日本医学英語教育学会・編

講義録
医学英語 II

科学英語への扉

編集　Nell L. Kennedy，菱田治子

Textbook of
English for
Medical Purposes
Volume II

Entering Scientific English in Context

MEDICAL VIEW

Textbook of English for Medical Purposes, Volume 2
Entering Scientific English in Context
ISBN 978–4–7583–0408–5 C3347

Edited by Nell L. Kennedy and Haruko Hishida
for the Japan Society for Medical English Education

2005. 12. 20   1st edition
2008. 2. 1   3rd printing

© MEDICAL VIEW, 2005, 2007, 2008
Printed and Bound in Japan

Medical View Co., Ltd.
2–30 Ichigaya–hommuracho, Shinjuku–ku, Tokyo 162–0845, Japan
E–mail   ed@medicalview.co.jp

刊行に寄せて

　本書は，医師・医療関係者に求められる英語力を総合的・体系的に習得するための全3巻の教科書として，日本医学英語教育学会により企画・編集されました。

　かねてから医師には英語力も必要だと言われていたものの，医師・医学生への英語教育は「医学」と「英語教育」という2つの異なる専門分野での知識が要求され，体系的に教育できるカリキュラムや教材もないまま，現場で担当する先生たちは独自の工夫をこらしつつ大変な努力をなさっていました。日本医学英語教育学会が1998年に設立された際には，その大きな目的の一つとして，この2つの分野の専門家たちが協力することによって，日本における医学英語教育の指針となるべき教科書を制作することがありました。爾来6年，その努力が実を結んだ成果が本書です。

　本書を企画段階において，医師に求められる英語力の到達目標として下記の3点が挙げられました。
  1. 英語で患者さんの診療を行える。
  2. 英語で医療・医学に関する発表・討論を行える。
  3. 英語で論文や書類を作成できる。

　最終的にこれらの目標に到達するためのステップとして，本書の各章は構成されています。全3巻は英語力の段階に応じて分けられており，初級向けの第1巻では語彙の充実や読解力の養成を，第2巻では医学の専門的内容にさらに踏み込んで症例報告や論文を題材として採り上げ，第3巻では実践の準備段階として，患者さんとの会話や口頭発表，論文執筆について学びます。

　言うまでもなく，外国語の習得に王道はありません。学生の間だけで上記の到達目標に到達するのは難しいかもしれませんが，卒業して医師となってからも，生涯続く英語学習の友として本書を活用していただければ，これに勝る喜びはありません。

　現在のわが国は，残念ながら諸外国からの評価としては「医学・医療知識の輸入国」としての地位に甘んじています。しかし前途有望な医師・医学生の皆さんが本書を学習の友として英語力の研鑚に励まれれば，その汚名を返上できる日も遠くはないと確信しています。

2004年12月

日本医学英語教育学会理事長
東京慈恵会医科大学脳神経外科教授
大井 静雄

序文

　第1巻『講義録　医学英語Ⅰ』に続いて，第2巻の刊行にあたりどのような教材が学習者に「医学英語」の特徴を伝えられるか，また「医学英語」を担当する先生方のニーズに応えられるか考えました。「医学英語」とは一般の英語と何が違うのでしょう。語彙が違うことは第1巻の専門用語で学びましたが，その他には？表現方法や科学的な論文の構成も一般の読みものとはかなり違います。学習者にはもちろん，医学を専門としない英語教師，あるいは逆に専門の英語表現に触れる機会が多く一般的な表現に馴染みの少ない医師にとっても必要な情報を盛り込んだ教材とはどのようなものか，いろいろ考えた末，一般の英語(general English)と科学/医学で使われる英語(scientific English)の違いを示すことをこの本の特徴にしました。したがって，この第2巻の前半の章はまず専門書ではなく TIME 誌や Voice of America(VOA)，National Public Radio(NPR)等の一般的なもののなかから医学に関連する題材を採り上げて，そのなかで科学英語との相違点を紹介し，後半の章では専門の論文，症例報告のなかで一般英語との相違点を示すように構成しました。

　　Chapters　1～3　：　一般誌の医学関連記事を読む
　　Chapters　4～6　：　一般の医学関連ニュースを聴き取る
　　Chapters　7～10：　医学論文の読み方
　　Chapters 11～12：　症例を読む

　各章には，学習者の理解を深めるために詳細な説明を加え，また学習を確実なものにするために練習問題をたくさん用意しました。しかし各章の練習問題は必ずしも全てをやっていただく必要はなく，このテキストを使用されるそれぞれの状況によって取捨選択していただければ結構です。
　後半の医学英語の専門に入って最初の医学論文の読み方の章では数ページにわたる英語の論文のポイントをごく短時間で把握できる方法がわかり，さらにそれが身につくよう練習問題が用意されています。学習者の皆さんにとってはもちろんですが，教師，医師の専門家にも大いに役立つと確信しています。この本で一般英語と科学英語/医学英語の違いを認識し，それが医学英語の理解をより深める一助になることを心から願っています。
　最後に，本書の発刊にあたり，辛抱強く見守り，編集・校正に多大な御尽力を頂きました日本医学英語教育学会事務局の江口潤司様に心より御礼申し上げます。

2005年11月

『講義録　医学英語Ⅱ』編集委員
浜松医科大学 総合人間科学講座(英語)

菱田　治子

To the Student

The main purpose of this book is to help you reach your goals. To get the most out of the book:

1. Listen to the CD over and over, with and without the text.
2. Ask yourself questions about the readings. For example:
   - In heart patients, do statins work better than surgery? Is aspirin better?
   - How can we reduce muscle injury in patients with McArdle's disease?
   - How can we prevent kidney failure in patients with McArdle's disease?
   - What made those doctors think about trying something as simple as oral sucrose?
   - As the first step in managing high blood pressure, are the new expensive drugs really better than a diuretic?
3. Write notes in the page margins, in English as much as possible.
4. When reading a passage the 2nd or 3rd time, cover the Japanese notes.
5. Number the points mentioned in series in the readings.
6. Look for opposing ideas.
7. Underline key points.
8. Look for patterns and relationships.
9. Go to the Web sites to see photographs and get more information.

Nell Kennedy, PhD
Professor, Biomedical English
School of Veterinary Medicine
Rakuno Gakuen University

Acknowledgments

We especially appreciate Prof. Toshio Ohki and Prof. Mitsuko Hirano for critically reading the book before and after publication and for giving concrete suggestions and prompt answers to our myriad of questions. We are indebted to Masahiko Motooka for making digital images of the editor's rough sketches of the coronary arteries and midsaggital sections of the midbrain and thalamus. We thank Masakazu Hirose and Daisuke Yokoyama for technical help and for advice on special expressions and Exercises. We are profoundly grateful to the 300 students or more who helped us test certain chapters and whose generous feedback was extremely helpful. And we owe a special debt of gratitude to Mr. Junji Eguchi, Secretariat for JASMEE and overseer of this project at the Digital Publishing Department, Medical View, for fine-tuning everything and turning chaos into order.

The Editors
Nell Kennedy and Haruko Hishida

Contents

刊行に寄せて … iii
序文 …………… iv
編集委員会 …… xii

Part 1　Reading Medical Features in News Magazines

Chapter 1　*What Is a Headache?*　2

Reading ─ 2
Word Study ─ 4
- migraineur … 4
- keeping their headaches at bay … 5
- biofeedback … 5

Grammatical Points ─ 6
- 倒置による，文の一部の強調（強調される語句が文頭に出てくるため語順が入れ替わる）… 6
- 過去分詞句，that 節がともに一つの名詞を修飾する … 6

Scientific English ─ 6
- トピック文（"umbrella sentence"）の順番とその後の説明の順番を一致させる … 6
- self-contained: 自己限定〔性〕の（self-limited）… 7

Exercises 1–5 ─ 8

Chapter 2　*The Migraine Mechanism*　12

Reading ─ 12
Grammatical Points ─ 14
- 先行詞と離れた that 節 … 14
- 動詞が 2 つの that 節を目的語としている … 14
- 不定詞：allow ... to ～（許可），cause ... to ～（原因）… 15

Scientific English ─ 15
- suggest の使い方 … 15

Exercises 1–5 ─ 16
Scientific English ─ 20
- Afferent nerves … 20
- Efferent nerves … 21

Exercise 6 ─ 21

Chapter 3　*Rethinking Treatments for the Heart*　22

Reading ———————————————————————————— 22
Word Study ————————————————————————— 25
- the best bet … 25
- fatty plaque, fatty deposit … 25

Scientific English ————————————————————— 25
- 短縮形（don't, isn't, can't, you'd） … 25
- 人称代名詞（they, you, we, them） … 25
- already … 26
- of course … 26
- seemed … 26
- 人以外の所有格 … 26

Exercises 1–7 ———————————————————————— 27

Part 2　Listening to Medical News Reports

Chapter 4　*Drugs for High Blood Pressure*　34

Exercises 1–8 ———————————————————————— 34
For Further Study ———————————————————— 38

Chapter 5　*The Battle between HIV and Antibodies*　40

Exercises 1–5 ———————————————————————— 40
For Further Study ———————————————————— 43

Chapter 6　*Drug to Stop Progression of Type 1 Diabetes*　46

Exercises 1–8 ———————————————————————— 46
For Further Study ———————————————————— 50

Part 3 Reading the Medical Research Paper

Chapter 7 *Entering the Medical Research Paper* 54

- **Lecture:** 医学論文入門 — 54
  - Title — 55
- **Exercises 1–2** — 56
- **Lecture:** What the Abstract can and cannot do 抄録の役割 — 57
  - **Reading warm-up:** The Effect of Oral Sucrose on Exercise Tolerance in Patients with McArdle's Disease — 58
    - ■ Abstract … 58
    - ■ Underline key words … 58
    - ■ Number the points from the known to the unknown … 58
- **Exercises 3–5** — 59
- **Lecture:** Pre-reading 準備体操 — 61
  - Entering the Main Body of the Paper — 61
  - The Research Problem — 62
- **Exercises 6–7** — 63
- **For Further Study:** Finding other papers and books for doctors Using the Internet to contact patients with McArdle's disease — 65

Chapter 8 *Reading the Introduction* 68
The Effect of Oral Sucrose on Exercise Tolerance in Patients with McArdle's Disease

- **Reading:** Introduction — 68
- **Lecture:** Clues and Patterns   A specific gap, or unknown, in medical knowledge is a clue to the authors' research aims — 70
- **Exercise 1** — 71
- **Lecture:** What kinds of information are usually in the Introduction? — 72
- **Exercises 2–4** — 72
- **Lecture:** Is the author's argument logical and convincing? — 76
- **Exercise 5** — 76
- **For Further Study:** See the sucrose drink — 77

Chapter 9 ***Methods · Results***　　78
The Effect of Oral Sucrose on Exercise Tolerance in Patients with McArdle's Disease

Reading: Methods	78
Lecture: Types of study designs	80

- single-blind（単盲検）… 80
- randomized（無作為化）… 81
- placebo-controlled（プラセボ対照）… 81
- crossover（クロスオーバー）… 81

Exercise 1 ——— 81

Lecture: What main information is in the Methods section?
　—Who, What, When, Where, How ——— 82

- WHO … 82
- WHAT … 82
- Approval by the Ethics Committee … 82
- Informed Consent … 83
- WHEN, WHERE, and HOW … 83
- Analysis … 83

Exercises 2–4 ——— 83

Reading: Results ——— 86

Lecture: What main information is in the Results section? ——— 88

- The bare data … 88
- Visual comparison … 88
- Statistics … 88

Exercises 5–8 ——— 88

For Further Study: A quick guide ——— 93

Chapter 10 ***Discussion***　　94
The Effect of Oral Sucrose on Exercise Tolerance in Patients with McArdle's Disease

Reading: Discussion ——— 94

Lecture: Clues to Reading the Discussion ——— 97

- 過去形の動詞 … 97
- 現在形の動詞 … 97

Exercises 1–2 ——— 98

Lecture:	What is the function of the Discussion?	100
	■ Discussion の役割 … 100	
	■ What questions should we ask? … 100	
Exercises 3–6		101
For Further Study		104
Exercises 7–8		105

Part 4 Reading the Case Report

Chapter 11 *Case Report: A 33-year-old Woman with Abdominal Pain, Vomiting, and Erythema* 108

Lecture:	The formal case report	108
Reading:	Case report	108
Lecture:	-ectomy / -tomy / -stomy	112
	Visual acuity: 視力の表記	112
	Prescriptions: 処方箋の書き方	113
	Third decade の和訳	113
	Percent of increase: ○%増加	113
Exercises 1–5		114
Lecture:	Why are 4 criteria necessary for a diagnosis of SLE?	119
Exercise 6		120
For Further Study:	I heard that foreign universities do not use ○ and ×. Is that true?	120
	What is the difference between an oral case report and a published case report?	121

Chapter 12 *Case Report: A 53-year-old Woman with Sudden Onset of Double Vision* 124

Reading:	Case report	124
Exercises 1–3		128
Lecture:	What can we expect from a Case Report?	131
	■ Key feature … 131	
	■ Message for the reader … 131	

- Message type A … 131
- Message type B … 131
- Chronological structure of published Case Reports … 132
- Do Case Reports count as research? … 132

Exercise 4 ───────────────────────────── **133**

Lecture: 「死亡する」という場合の前置詞 ─────── **134**

    Two or more と more than two ────────── **134**

    人名の発音 ─────────────────── **134**

Exercises 5–6 ───────────────────────── **135**

Appendix: Training to Listen like a Scientist

    In search of clinical evidence　臨床的根拠の探求 ── **137**

Index ────────────────────────── **140**

COLUMNS

- VOA Special English について ……………………………… 39
- VOA News について ……………………………………… 44
- NPR について ……………………………………………… 51
- お薦めのリスニング・インターネット無料サイト …………… 52
- Informal Messages from Patients with McArdle's Disease … 66
- Finding the Unknown …………………………………… 77
- Autosomal Recessive Genetic Disorder ………………… 102
- Specializing ……………………………………………… 122

日本医学英語教育学会
医学英語教科書編集委員会

■編集委員会

小林充尚（委員長）	防衛医科大学校名誉教授
大木俊夫	浜松医科大学名誉教授
大武　博	京都府立医科大学第一外国語教室教授
大野典也	東京慈恵会医科大学名誉教授
Nell L. Kennedy	酪農学園大学獣医学部バイオメディカルイングリッシュ研究室教授
清水雅子	川崎医療福祉大学英語教授
羽白　清	元・京都大学
J. Patrick Barron	東京医科大学国際医学情報センター教授
菱田治子	聖路加看護大学　教養・英語　教授

■第2巻担当編集委員

Nell L. Kennedy	酪農学園大学獣医学部バイオメディカルイングリッシュ研究室教授
菱田治子	聖路加看護大学　教養・英語　教授

■第2巻執筆者

名木田恵理子	川崎医療短期大学教授（Chapters 1～3）
内藤　永	旭川医科大学医学部英語助教授（Chapter 4～6）
Nell L. Kennedy	酪農学園大学獣医学部バイオメディカルイングリッシュ研究室教授（Chapters 7～10）
菱田治子	聖路加看護大学　教養・英語　教授（Chapters 7～10）
大石　実	日本大学練馬光が丘病院神経内科助教授（Chapters 11～12）

Part 1
Reading Medical Features in News Magazines

Part 1: Reading Medical Features in News Magazines

Chapter 1 What Is a Headache?

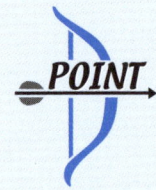

医科学系の文は，文学作品などの文と異なり，文法の基本に忠実で明瞭な構造をもっているのが一般的です。そのような文では，主語，述語，目的語をつかめばおおむね文意を把握することができます。この Chapter では，まず正確に客観的に意味をとっていくことから始めましょう。

Reading CD

CD track 1

1　First, let's define a few terms. Doctors divide headaches into two broad categories: those that are self-contained (primary headaches) and those that result from another illness or accident (secondary
5　headaches). The best treatment for a secondary headache depends on its origin. For example, an antibiotic may be prescribed for a headache caused by a bacterial infection.

　The most common type of primary headache is the
10　familiar tension headache, which is usually stress related. (Doctors now label it a tension-type headache.) In most cases, a couple of aspirin and a good night's sleep are all that's required to get rid of one.

　Not so the mercifully uncommon cluster headache,
15　so named because an attack typically repeats itself, often daily, with each episode lasting anywhere from an hour to an hour and a half. Cluster headaches usually strike their victims, generally men, at fixed times of the

self-contained: 自己限定〔性〕の（= self-limited）

primary: 原発の，一義的な

antibiotic: 抗生物質

prescribe: 処方する

bacterial infection: 細菌感染症

tension: 緊張

cluster headache: 群発性頭痛

attack: 発作，突発的症状の発現

episode: 症状の発現（持続する病気の経過中に起こる単一あるいは一連の症状発現）

year. The pain is so searing that they are also known as suicide headaches. Immediate treatment with oxygen and migraine drugs given intravenously can sometimes provide relief.

Somewhere between tension and cluster headaches are migraines. Typically, the pain from a migraine is a throbbing one, restricted to one side of the head, that gets worse with movement and lasts from four hours to three days. Migraines are usually accompanied by either nausea and vomiting or extreme sensitivity to both light and sound. By contrast, patients suffering from tension-type headaches may react badly to either light or sound but not both.

It is a mistake, however, to stick too rigidly to these definitions. At one time people thought that migraine was a disorder all its own and that tension-type headache was totally separate. Researchers now realize that headaches are not that clear cut. Nearly any recurring headache that is debilitating enough to keep you away from work or the things you enjoy is probably a migraine.

Ideally, you'd like to prevent a migraine from occurring in the first place. There is a lot you can do to help yourself. Identifying individual triggers—such as chocolate or fluorescent lights—and keeping away from them as much as possible is an obvious first step. You should also avoid relying too heavily on quick fixes. People with severe migraine headaches can enter a cycle of taking medications on a daily or near daily basis. Initially it helps, but over time the headaches get worse.

Many migraineurs swear by various nonpharmacological methods of keeping their headaches at bay, such as yoga, meditation and biofeedback. These techniques probably work best for patients whose headaches are triggered by stress or tense facial muscles.

It may be still a process of trial and error for most patients and their physicians. Chances are, however, that more and more of them will eventually hit on the combination of medications and lifestyle changes that works for them.

Excerpt from "The New Science of Headaches," by Christine Gorman and Alice Park. *Time*. October 7, 2002, Asian edition. Used with permission and special courtesy of TIME Inc.

migraineur, at bay: see pp. 4–5, Word Study
swear by ...: …に頼りきる
nonpharmacological: 非薬物の
yoga: ヨガ
meditation: 瞑想
biofeedback: see p. 5, Word Study
chances are that ...: おそらく

line 50

Word Study

● **migraineur**

　TIME の記事では「片頭痛患者」を，migraine sufferer, victim, patient と表していますが，同時に migraineur という語も使っています。migraine はもともとフランス語（さらにさかのぼればギリシャ語の hemi-（半分）＋ cranium（頭蓋骨）に由来する）からの借用語です。migraineur は migraine に -eur という「ある行動をする人，ある働きをする道具」などの意味をもつフランス語の接尾辞がついたものです。他にもこういった類いの語には，provocateur（警察のおとり），voyeur（のぞき趣味の人），connoisseur（美術品の鑑定家）などがあります。

　sufferer という語には，その意味から「かわいそうな被害者」という感情的なセンセーショナルな響きがあります。ジャーナリズムでは，感情過剰な語をなるべく使わないという原則があります。そのため，*TIME* では migraineurs を使っているのでしょう。

● **keeping their headaches at bay**

　興味深い表現です。この場合の bay は「獲物を追いつめていくときの猟犬の吠え声」のこと。そのことから「獣や逃亡者などを吠えて食い止める」という意味が生まれています。keep an enemy at bay（敵を食い止める），have a bear at bay（熊を追いつめて逃さない）などの表現があります。

　TIME の記事では migraine を「敵」や「危険な獣」として比喩しています。

line 51

● **biofeedback**

　そもそも feedback とは，「あることに対して返される反応」という意味です。学生にとって試験を受けてその成績が返されるのは，一種の feedback です。学生はそれによって自分がどの程度学んだのかを知ることができます。

　それを生体について行うのが，biofeedback（生体自己防御）です。つまり，からだに取り付けられた器械（筋電図計，血圧計，脳波，心電図計など）が表す数値，グラフによって，自分のからだの中の状態を知ることができるのです。

　これが特にストレス緩和の手段として使われています。患者は数値やグラフを見ることによって，自分のからだをコントロールする方法を覚えます。例えば，筋肉の緊張の度合いを筋電図で知り，どういうふうにしたら落ち着いた状態になるかを体得していくのです。

line 52

Grammatical Points

1. 倒置による，文の一部の強調（強調される語句が文頭に出てくるため語順が入れ替わる）

   - Not so the mercifully uncommon cluster headache, so named because an attack typically repeats itself, often daily, with each episode lasting anywhere from an hour to an hour and a half.　　　lines 14–17

     ありがたいことに一般的でない型の群発型頭痛ではそうはいかない。（アスピリンを飲んでよく眠れば治るというわけにはいかない。）この頭痛は発作が毎日のように繰り返され，毎回の発作が1時間から1時間半続くのが典型で，そのように名づけられている。

   - Somewhere between tension and cluster headaches are migraines.　　　lines 23–24

     片頭痛は，緊張型と群発型の間に位置している。

2. 過去分詞句，that 節がともに一つの名詞を修飾する

   - ... a throbbing one, restricted to one side of the head, that gets worse with movement and lasts from four hours to three days.　　　lines 24–27

     頭の片方に限局していて，動くと悪化し，4時間から3日間も続く，ズキンズキンという痛み

Scientific English

科学英語：ここが違う！

トピック文（"umbrella sentence"）の順番とその後の説明の順番を一致させる

　　TIME の記事の最初の段落では，2番目の文で primary　　　lines 3, 4

headachesとsecondary headachesが，この順番で述べられていますが，その後の文章では，secondary headachesのほうがprimary headachesよりも先に説明されています。しかし，医学雑誌では，トピックとして示される順番と，その後の説明の順番は常に同じです。説明の順番を同じにできないのであれば，トピックとして示す順番を変えなくてはなりません。そうでなければ，読者は混乱し，時間を無駄にしてしまいます。科学研究論文では，順番が著者と読者を結ぶ大事な手がかりなのです。

lines 5, 9

> 科学英語：ここが違う！

self-contained: 自己限定〔性〕の（self-limited）

このTIMEではself-containedはself-limited（自己限定性の）と同意のように使われています。科学英語では"self-limited"（まれに"self-limiting"）と説明される疾患があります。以下はThe New England Journal of Medicineで使われている例です。

line 3

Mondor's disease is characterized by thrombophlebitis of the subcutaneous veins of the anterolateral thoracoabdominal wall. The condition is three times as frequent in women as in men and is usually benign and **self-limited**. Our patient was given nonsteroidal antiinflammatory drugs. The lesion and pain both **disappeared within six weeks**, and the patient has subsequently been well. [*N Engl J Med* 2005; 352:1024]

［訳］モンドール病は，胸腹壁前外側の皮下静脈における血栓性静脈炎を特徴とする。本疾患は男性よりも女性に3倍多く発症し，通常は良性かつ自己限定性である。著者らが担当した患者は非ステロイド抗炎症薬を投与された。病変および痛みはともに6週間以内に消失し，その後も患者の状態は良好である。

TIMEでは"an epidemic is difficult to contain"のように"to contain"を"to limit"の意味で使ってしまったり，一人の教員がすべての教科を担当する小学校のクラスを"self-contained"と言ったり，表現を創作することがよくあります。

TIMEの読者はこのような言い方に慣れているので，primary headacheが"self-contained"であるといえば，他の条件によらないそれ単独の頭痛だということがわかります。

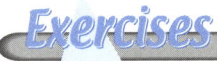

1. **Vocabulary**

    英文の説明に該当する語を右の囲みから選んで書きなさい。

_____	1. a kind of medicine that inhibits the growth of microorganisms	an antibiotic
_____	2. a doctor's written instruction for the use of a medicine or treatment	an attack
		an episode
_____	3. an event occurring as part of a sequence	eventually
_____	4. into a vein	a fix
_____	5. sick feeling with inclination to vomit	intravenous
_____	6. the quality of responding rapidly to some stimulus, such as to a chemical or light	medication
		nausea
_____	7. to cause something to happen	a prescription
_____	8. a medicine or drug	sensitivity
_____	9. a dose of a narcotic drug, which can cause addiction	trigger
		vomiting
_____	10. ultimately	

2. **Summing Up**

    それぞれの（　）内の定義に従い，頭痛を分類しなさい。

    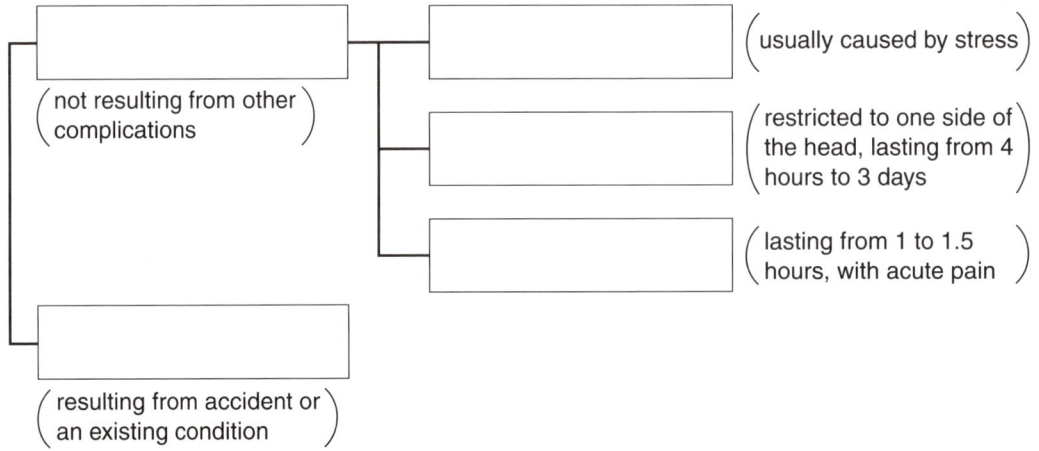

3. Scanning

Reading の内容に沿って英文を完成させなさい。

1. There are two types of headaches. One is a ① _____ headache, and the other is a ② _____ ③ _____ , which is sequential to another illness or an ④ _____ and can be managed by treating its ⑤ _____ .

2. The tension headache, referred to as a ⑥ _____ headache, is often related to ⑦ _____ . Usually the pain can be relieved by taking ⑧ _____ and getting enough ⑨ _____ .

3. In a cluster headache, an ⑩ _____ repeats itself and the pain is severe. The victims of cluster headaches are generally ⑪ _____ .

4. The migraine headache, which is restricted to one side of the ⑫ _____ , is often accompanied by ⑬ _____ and ⑭ _____ . Some persons with a migraine may also experience extreme ⑮ _____ to light and sound.

5. To prevent a migraine, it is necessary to ⑯ _____ individual triggers and ⑰ _____ away from them.

6. Some medications are helpful, but you should avoid ⑱ _____ too much on them. Instead, you can make use of various methods such as yoga, ⑲ _____ and ⑳ _____ .

4. Composition. A Short Summary

Reading で採り上げた記事の Summary をつくりましょう。科学英語の書き方 (p. 6) を参考に，枠内の 5 つの英文から 3 つを選び，論理的な流れに沿って順序よくその 3 つの英文を続けて書きなさい。

> The secondary headache mentioned in the article is one caused by a bacterial infection.
>
> This article describes three types of primary headache and mentions one type of secondary headache.
>
> The primary headaches described are the cluster, migraine and tension-type headaches.
>
> The primary headaches described are the tension-type, cluster and migraine headaches.
>
> The primary headaches described are the tension-type, migraine and cluster headaches.

_____

_____

_____

_____

_____

_____

Checkpoint 多くの学生が，tension と書くべきところを誤って tention と書き，また migraine を migrain と書いてしまいます。あなたはどうですか？

5. 科学英語 Composition: Comparing

　Tension-type headache と migraine headache の光と音に対する感受性に関連する違いは何ですか。この質問に対する答えを下記の単語をすべて使って，2 つの英文として書きなさい。×2 となっている単語は 2 回使います。

注意：トピック文（umbrella sentence）での順番に従って書きましょう。また文の最初の単語
　　　は大文字で始め，句読点を適切なところに入れなさい。

a migraine headache	either	people (×2)
a tension-type headache	extremely	sensitive (×2)
and	light (×2)	sound (×2)
are (×2)	not	to (×2)
both (×1 or ×2)	on the other hand	who have (×2)
but	or	

_____

_____

_____

_____

_____

Part 1: Reading Medical Features in News Magazines

Chapter 2 The Migraine Mechanism

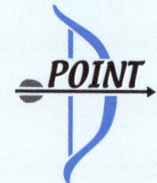

POINT 文が集まって文章が組み立てられます。内容を正しく「読解」するには，一つ一つの文の意味を解読するだけでは不十分で，文の流れに沿って話の筋道をつかんでいくことが要求されます。それには文と文とをつなぐ副詞（句）や接続詞もヒントになります。これらを道標にして話の筋道を追っていきましょう。

Reading

CD track 2

1   As far back as the 1600s, the prominent English physician Thomas Willis suggested that headaches are caused by a rapid increase in the flow of blood to the brain. He theorized that the suddenly bulging blood
5   vessels put pressure on nearby nerves and that these in turn trigger the pain. A variation on Willis' idea became the favored explanation for the cause of migraines. (An important network of blood vessels at the base of the brain bears Willis' name.)

10   Two things have occurred in the past couple of decades to alter that view. First, several imaging techniques were developed that allowed doctors to study blood flow in the living brain. Second, scientists learned a great deal more about the nerve endings that
15   are embedded in the dura mater, the fibrous outer covering of the brain. Armed with these tools and that information, researchers concluded that the order of events in a migraine is not as straightforward as they

prominent: 卓越した

bulge: ふくらむ
blood vessel: 血管
nerve: 神経

imaging technique: 造影技術

nerve ending:〔軸索の〕神経終末

embed: ぴったりとはめ込む

dura mater:〔脳・脊髄の〕硬膜 [djύərə méitə(r)]

fibrous: 線維 (fiber) の

had been taught. The nerve endings in the dura mater appear to act first, releasing proteins that cause the blood vessels to open and prime the nerves to maintain a state of alert. In other words, swollen blood vessels are the result of a growing migraine, not its cause.

Tracing the pathway of the affected nerve endings deeper into the brain led researchers to the trigeminal nerve, a complex network of nerve fibers that ferries sensory signals from the face, jaws and top of the forehead to the brain. During the course of a migraine, scientists discovered, the trigeminal nerve practically floods the brain with pain signals. The more researchers learn about the trigeminal nerve, the more they believe that it is involved in all types of primary headaches, including tension and cluster headaches. The differences in the headache types seem to stem from what activates the trigeminal nerve and how it responds.

So much is happening all at once during a migraine that it has been hard to pinpoint what sets off the trigeminal nerve. Some scientists are focusing on a wave of electrical activity that spreads across the brain just before a migraine and triggers the aura—the shimmering light show experienced by 1 in 5 migraine patients. Others wonder whether there is some kind of migraine generator buried deep within the brain stem. Even when researchers think they know the order in which different parts of the brain turn on during an attack, they can't always be sure if one section is initiating an action or anticipating the need to respond.

What seems clear, however, is that the brain of a migraineur is primed to overreact to all sorts of stimuli that most people can easily tolerate. The brain receives input from a wide variety of triggers—stress, hormones, falling barometric pressure, food, drink, sleep disturbances. Each of us has his own stack of triggers and his own personal threshold at which the migraine mechanism activates. The higher the trigger level climbs above the threshold, the more fully activated the migraine system—and the more pain.

In this view, people who are prone to migraine have a low threshold for activating the trigeminal nerve. Those who suffer only an occasional tension-type headache have a much higher threshold. Persistent treatment of acute attacks and prevention of additional ones may reset the brain's threshold point at a higher level.

Excerpt from "The New Science of Headaches," by Christine Gorman and Alice Park. *Time*. October 7, 2002, Asian edition. Used with permission and special courtesy of TIME Inc.

hormone: ホルモン [hɔ́ərmoun | hɔ́ː-]

barometric pressure: 気圧

stack of: たくさんの

threshold: 閾値（刺激を感知しはじめる点） (see p. 96 line 50)

(be) prone to ...: 〔通常は悪いことで〕…の傾向がある (see p. 70 line 49)

persistent: 持続的な

Grammatical Points

1. **先行詞と離れた that 節**
   - ... several imaging techniques were developed **that** allowed doctors to study blood flow ...

   医師が血流の研究をするのを可能にしたいくつかの造影技術が開発された（that 節の先行詞は imaging techniques）

   lines 11–13

2. **動詞が 2 つの that 節を目的語としている**
   - He theorized **that** the suddenly bulging blood vessels put pressure on nearby nerves and **that** these in turn trigger the pain.

   彼は，急に拡張した血管が付近の神経を圧迫し，次にそれが痛

   lines 4–6

みを誘発するという理論を立てた。

3．不定詞：allow ... to 〜（可能），cause ... to 〜（原因）
- First, several imaging techniques were developed that **allowed** doctors **to** study blood flow in the living brain.　　lines 11–13

  1つには，生きた脳における血流を医師が研究できる造影技術がいくつか開発された。

- ... releasing proteins that **cause** the blood vessels **to** open　　lines 21–22

  …蛋白を放出し，それが血管を開かせる

Scientific English

科学英語：ここが違う！

suggest の使い方
- 一般英語：人（主語）＋ **suggest**
- 科学英語：原理・原則（主語）＋ **suggest**

TIME が掲載する "The Migraine Mechanism" のような医学記事では，読みやすい会話体の文章と専門的な英語表現や用語がうまく合わさって特徴的な文体をつくっています。この "ハイブリッド" 方式は専門家だけでなく，専門知識に乏しい数百万人の一般読者にもとても人気があります。しかし，医学専門誌では文体が *TIME* とはかなり異なっています。

- 一般英語：　Thomas Willis <u>suggested</u> that headaches are caused by a rapid increase in the flow of blood to the brain.　　line 2

- 科学英語：　Thomas Willis <u>proposed/advocated/suspected/maintained/conjectured/believed</u> that ...

- 違いは何?：「人 ＋ suggest」は会話でよく使われる表現です（例：My teacher suggested that I enter this university.）。しかし科学専門誌の編集者たち

はこの形を好みません。科学英語では，suggest はほとんどの場合，データや科学的な解釈・判断，報告等，人以外の語を主語としています。

Exercises

1. **Vocabulary**

   英文の説明に該当する語を右の囲みから選んで書きなさい。

   _____ 1. distinguished, renowned

   _____ 2. a duct or canal conveying blood or other fluid

   _____ 3. consisting of fibers

   _____ 4. a device, typically hand-held

   _____ 5. to set free

   _____ 6. to keep a condition at the same level or rate

   _____ 7. a thing that evokes a specific functional reaction

   _____ 8. a substance produced by a living organism

   _____ 9. to convert a substance into a reactive form

   _____ 10. the point at which an event or effect starts to take place in response to a stimulus

   activate
   fibrous
   generate
   hormone
   maintain
   meditation
   prominent
   relieve
   stimulus
   threshold
   tool
   vessel

2. **Comprehension**

   日本語で答えなさい。

   1. Willis は頭痛の原因をどう説明しましたか。

2. Willis の説に修正を加えるきっかけを与えた2つのこととは何ですか。

   _____

3. その結果，頭痛はどのようにして起こると説明されましたか。

   _____

4. 頭痛が起こっている間，三叉神経はどのように反応していますか。

   _____

5. 頭痛が起こるのに個人差があるのはなぜですか。

   _____

3. Summing Up: 頭痛のメカニズム

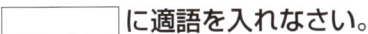に適語を入れなさい。

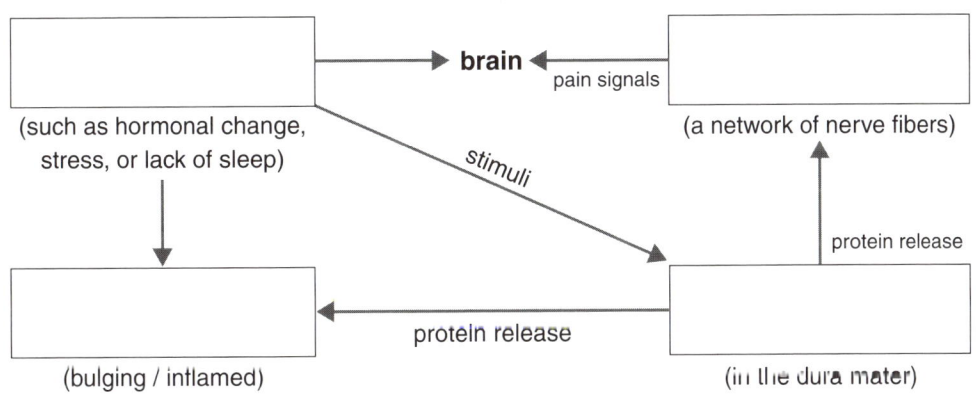

4. Scanning

Reading の内容に沿って英文を完成させなさい。

1. A 17th-century English doctor, Thomas Willis, theorized the headache mechanism as follows: a rapid ① _____ in blood flow to the brain causes the blood

vessels to become so full that they put ② _____ on nearby nerves and these nerves then trigger the ③ _____ that we refer to as a headache.

2. Around 20 years ago, thanks to the development of ④ _____ ⑤ _____ and to information about the nerve endings in the ⑥ _____ , researchers have changed their view on the causes of headaches. They now believe that the nerve endings act first, releasing ⑦ _____ that cause the blood ⑧ _____ to open and stimulate the nerves to maintain a state of ⑨ _____ .

3. During the course of a migraine, the trigeminal nerve sends many ⑩ _____ ⑪ _____ to the brain. The trigeminal nerve appears to be involved in all types of ⑫ _____ headaches, including ⑬ _____ and ⑭ _____ headaches.

4. The brain receives input from a wide variety of ⑮ _____ , such as stress and sleep ⑯ _____ . In a person prone to migraine, the brain tends to overreact to all sorts of ⑰ _____ . In other words, the person's ⑱ _____ at which the migraine mechanism activates is lower than that of most people.

5. About ⑲ _____ percent of migraine patients experience an ⑳ _____ , or shimmering light, just before the migraine strikes.

5. Usage Awareness: 科学英語

例に示したように，それぞれの英文から主語と動詞を抜き出して下線部に書きなさい。また元の文章では，主部全体に下線を，また動詞に二重下線を引きなさい。

例：It is difficult to make predictions regarding the resurgence of SARS, but the current information suggests that the greatest risk of re-emergence of the disease may derive from an animal reservoir or infections transmitted in the laboratory.

　information suggests

1. Our findings suggest that coronary-artery atherosclerosis is more prevalent among patients with lupus than in the general population. (Asanuma Yu, Oeser Annette et al. 2003. Premature coronary-artery atherosclerosis in systemic lupus erythematosus. *N Engl J Med* 349: 2407–2414.)

2. The lack of awareness of these hazards on the part of both the public and some physicians suggests the need for greater education. (Schiodt, Frank V. et al. 1997. Acetaminophen toxicity in an urban county hospital. *N Engl J Med* 338: 1112–1118.)

3. A review of the data suggests that SARS–CoV may be far more stable than the other human respiratory viruses.

4. The estimated time between the exposure to poultry and the onset of illness suggests an incubation period of two to four days. (Hien, Tran Tinh et al. 2004. Avian influenza A [H5N1] in 10 patients in Vietnam. *N Engl J Med* 350: 1179–1188.)

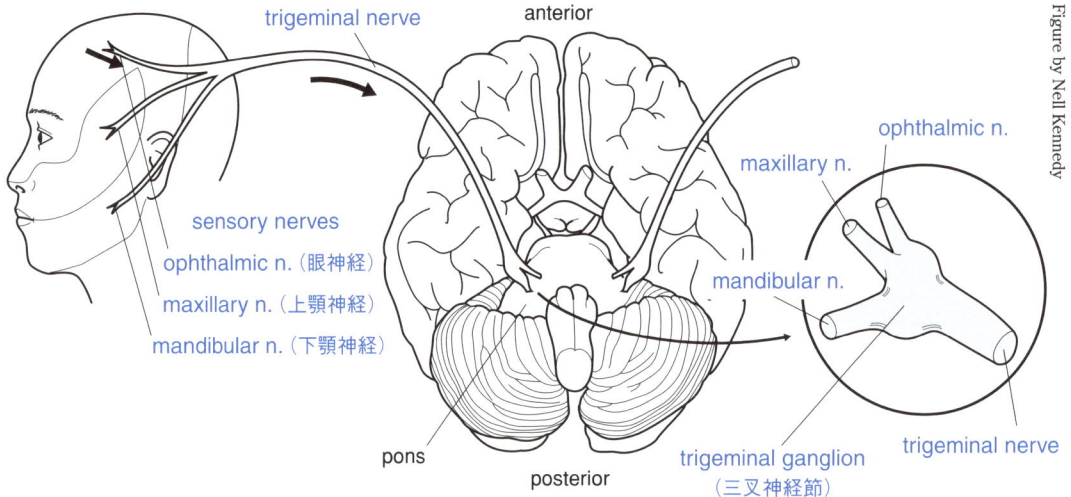

Figure 2.1. Sensory portions of the trigeminal nerve.

The trigeminal nerve, i.e., cranial nerve V, is the largest of the 12 pairs of cranial nerves. The three sensory branches, converging in the pons, are the ophthalmic n., maxillary (upper jaw) n., and mandibular (lower jaw) n. The ophthalmic n. contains fibers from the skin over the anterior half of the scalp, forehead, upper eyelid, eyeball, lacrimal glands, nasal cavity, and side of the nose. When migraines occur, the ophthalmic n. notifies the brain by conveying sensations of pain from the anterior half of the scalp and the forehead. The motor nerves are not shown in this figure.

三叉神経の感覚部.

三叉神経，すなわち第Ⅴ脳神経は，12対の脳神経中最も大きなものである。脳橋に集まる3つの感覚枝は眼神経，上顎神経，下顎神経である。眼神経は前頭部の頭皮，前額部，上眼瞼，眼球，涙腺，鼻腔，鼻部の皮膚からの線維を含む。片頭痛が起こるときは，眼神経が前頭部の頭皮と前額部からの痛覚を脳へ伝達する。この図に運動神経は示してありません。

Scientific English

科学英語：ここが違う！

... a complex <u>network</u> of nerve fibers that **ferries** sensory signals from the face, jaws and top of the forehead to the brain

p. 13, lines 27–29

■ Afferent nerves

An **afferent nerve** carries a message **to** or **toward** the brain or spinal cord but does not relay the response from the brain. In Latin, *af (ad)* means "to" or "toward," as in *adjuvant therapy, adhere, advance*. Thus, *af-* (to) + *ferent* (to carry, to ferry) = *afferent* (to carry to, to carry toward). However, several readers of this feature story have mistaken "ferries" to mean "to and fro" in lines 27–29, because the

afferent: 求心性の
relay: 中継する
adjuvant therapy: 補助療法 [ǽdʒʊvənt]
adhere (= stick to): 付着する
advance: move toward

dictionary lists "back and forth" as one of the meanings of "ferry." The direction of messages carried by afferent nerves is shown by arrows in Fig. 2.1. "To ferry" is a useful verb <u>for doctor-to-patient communication</u> if we explain that this nerve is a one-way ferry.

"ferry" はここでは一方向のみの意味

■ Efferent nerves

The nerves that move **out** from, or **away from**, the brain or spinal cord are the **efferent nerves**. *Ef-* (ex-, out) + *fer-rent* (to carry, to ferry) = *efferent* (to carry out of, to carry away from). The mandibular nerve has an afferent portion (Fig. 2.1) as well as an efferent portion (not shown in Fig. 2.1). <u>For doctor-to-staff communication</u>, the medical terms *afferent* and *efferent* help reduce ambiguity and make sure the meaning is crystal clear.

efferent: 遠心性の

mandibular: 下顎の

ambiguity: あいまいさ

Exercise

6. Working with afferent and efferent nerves

下の枠内から最適と思われる語を 1 つずつ選び，下線部に書き込みなさい。

1. The medical term for a sensory nerve is _____ nerve.

2. The medical term for a motor nerve is _____ nerve.

3. Efferent nerves carry messages _____ .

4. Afferent nerves carry messages _____ .

5. An _____ nerve tells the lower jaw to move or chew.

6. An _____ nerve relays a headache message from the scalp to the brain.

| afferent | efferent | to the brain | away from the brain | to and from the brain |

Part 1: Reading Medical Features in News Magazines

Chapter 3 Rethinking Treatments for the Heart

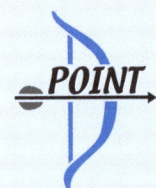

文章は，いくつかのパラグラフ（段落）に分けられます。パラグラフはそれぞれ一つの主題を展開し，そして各パラグラフが階層構造をつくって，全体を構成しているのです。まず，パラグラフの主題は何かをつかむことを心がけましょう。多くの場合，主題は各パラグラフの第一文に書かれています。そして，全体を論理的に読み取っていきましょう。

Reading

1　　For decades surgery seemed to be the best bet for the treatment of heart disease. Researchers thought of atherosclerosis, or the clogging of arteries with fatty plaques, as basically a plumbing problem. Bypass the
5　choke points with new grafts and you would more than likely bypass any future heart attacks. Over the past five to 10 years, however, doctors have come to realize that heart disease is more complicated than that. They're not by any means ready to abandon surgery,
10　but now they rely more heavily on different types of drugs to treat both the long-term and short-term effects of heart disease.

　　Drugs will play an even greater role in the near future. For one thing, the wealth of data coming out of
15　the human-genome project will allow physicians to tailor pharmaceutical treatments to an individual's specific genetic profile in ways that have never before been pos-

CD track 3
surgery: 手術
best bet: 最善の選択（see p. 25）
atherosclerosis: アテローム性動脈硬化症
clog: 血管を詰まらせる
plaque: 斑，プラーク（アテローム性の硬化病変部）（see p. 25）
a plumbing problem: 排水管の問題（ここでは血管の血流のこと）
bypass: バイパスを形成する，回避する
graft: 接ぎ木，移植片（ここでは代用血管のこと）
not by any means = by no means（決して〜でない）
rely on: …に頼る
human-genome: ヒトゲノム　[dʒíːnoum]
tailor ... to 〜: …を〜に合わせる
pharmaceutical treatment: 薬物治療
genetic: 遺伝子の

sible. For another, men and women at risk of developing heart disease are being identified at earlier and earlier stages of their condition, a situation in which drug therapy presents fewer risks than surgery.

To get a better idea of what could be in store, it helps to know what physicians believe lies at the root of most heart attacks. The trouble begins decades earlier, when the inside of a coronary artery becomes damaged—usually as a result of chronic high blood pressure, high cholesterol or the deleterious effects of smoking. The body tries to repair the damage, and a kind of internal scab is formed. Years go by, and the scab develops into a fatty deposit, filled with cholesterol, proteins and bits of cellular detritus. Sometimes the plaque is quite stable, and nothing much happens. Other times, for reasons that are still unclear, it becomes inflamed and prone to rupture. If the plaque breaks open, a clot forms, choking off the supply of blood. If the interruption lasts long enough, a heart attack ensues.

Doctors have already shown that drugs called statins, which curb the body's ability to manufacture excess cholesterol, can significantly reduce the risk of a heart attack. But statins don't work for everyone. So drug companies are studying the biochemical pathways by which the body pulls cholesterol that has already been manufactured out of a cell. By turning this reverse cholesterol transport on, you'd be able to stimulate removal of cholesterol from vessel walls back to the liver for excretion.

Researchers are also searching for new drugs to

dampen the inflammation process. The goal of such treatments is not so much to remove a fatty plaque from inside an artery but rather to convert it from a more dangerous form to a more stable one. This may be one of the reasons a daily dose of aspirin, which is both an anti-inflammatory and a blood thinner, can help prevent heart attacks. But doctors would like to have a drug that targets coronary inflammation more specifically and aggressively than aspirin.

There's more to heart disease, of course, than heart attacks. More and more Americans are developing a condition called congestive heart failure, in which the cardiac muscle becomes weakened and can no longer pump blood efficiently. Investigators are currently studying a group of specialized hormones that are released whenever the heart muscle falters. Some of these hormones help restore the heart's vigor while others, paradoxically, make the muscle stiffer and more difficult to contract. The goal is to figure out a way to boost the levels of the beneficial hormones while lowering those that make the weakened heart's job more difficult.

Of course, there would be much less need for new medications to treat heart disease if we all exercised more, watched our weight and stopped eating so much food that is high in saturated fat. Public-health experts estimate that you can reduce your risk of heart disease as much as 80% by adopting a healthy lifestyle.

Excerpt from "Rethinking Treatments for the Heart," by Christine Gorman. *Time.* January 22, 2001, Asian edition. Used with permission and special courtesy of TIME Inc.

---

dampen: 低下させる

anti-inflammatory:
抗炎症薬（ハイフンなしで antiinflammatory とも書く。see p. 7, Mondor's disease, line 5. また，この言葉は形容詞［抗炎症の］としても使われる）

congestive heart failure: うっ血性心不全

cardiac muscle: 心筋

paradoxically: 逆説的に

figure out: 考え出す

medication: see p. 3, line 47

saturated fat: 飽和脂肪

as much as: 〜もの

Word Study

● **the best bet**

bet には「賭け」「賭けの対象となる人，あるいは物」という意味がありますが，ここでの意味は「選択(choice)」です。ただしこの表現は口語的で，研究論文などにはふさわしくありません。"the best choice" という表現のほうが適切です。

line 1

● **fatty plaque, fatty deposit**

ここでの fat は「脂肪」という意味，fatty は「脂肪の，脂肪分を(多量に)含む」という意味です。血管に堆積する fatty plaque や fatty deposit は，中性脂肪(triglyceride)ばかりでなく，他の脂質(lipids)も混じっています。例えば，コレステロール(cholesterol)やリン脂質(phospholipid)，脂肪酸(fatty acid)，飽和脂肪(saturated fat)など。

lines 4, 30, 32, 34

Scientific English

科学英語：ここが違う！

以下に示した1～6の項目は，一般英語では日常的に使われますが，科学英語ではここに示したような表現のほうが適切です。

1．短縮形（don't, isn't, can't, you'd）

・一般英語：statins <u>don't work</u> for everyone

・科学英語：statins <u>are contraindicated</u> in some cases

line 41

contraindicated: 禁忌である（contra- [against / opposite] + indicate [to point]）

2．人称代名詞（they, you, we, them）

・一般英語：<u>They're not by any means ready</u> to abandon surgery, but now <u>they</u> rely more heavily on ...

lines 9–10

- ・科学英語： Although surgery is still a treatment option, drugs <u>are proving effective</u> for treating both the long-term and short-term effects of heart disease.

- ・一般英語： By turning this reverse cholesterol transport on, <u>you'd be able to</u> stimulate ...   lines 44–45
- ・科学英語： This reverse cholesterol transport would stimulate ...

3．already
- ・一般英語： Doctors have <u>already</u> shown that drugs called statins ...   line 38
- ・科学英語： Statins have been reported to ... / Statins are known to ...

4．of course
- ・一般英語： <u>There's more to</u> heart disease, <u>of course</u>, than heart attacks.   line 58
- ・科学英語： Heart disease encompasses not only heart attacks.

5．seemed
- ・一般英語： ... <u>seemed to be</u> the best bet for the treatment   line 1
- ・科学英語： ... was considered the treatment of choice for heart disease / was deemed ... / was by consensus the best ... / was believed to be the best ...

6．人以外の所有格
- ・一般英語： ... restore the <u>heart's</u> vigor ...   line 65
- ・科学英語： ... restore the <u>vigor of the heart</u>

一般英語は，ディスカッションや会話に向いています。聴き手はわからないことを質問できますし，話し手は口調や表情によって微妙な表現に明確な意味を与え，また要点を強調することもできます。ところが学術論文では，they や it, them といった代名詞が何を指しているのかが曖昧だと，誤解を招く原因となります。it が指しているのは治療なのか，症状なのか，決定したことなのか，数量なのか。they が指しているのは医師なのか，それとも薬物なのか。seemed はどの程度の確実性を意味しているのか。

　もちろん医学専門誌でも，TIME で使われているような一般英語を時折使うことは許されていますし，一般英語と科学英語の間に明確な境界線があるわけではありません。ただ，一般的に科学英語は TIME と比べると，"There is"で始まる文は少なく，ジャーナルを正確に読まなければならない科学者のために，曖昧さのない文章でなければなりません。

Exercises

1. **Vocabulary**

   英文の説明に該当する語を右の囲みから選んで書きなさい。

_____	1. an operation
_____	2. fatty substance present in most body tissues
to _____	3. to break or burst suddenly
_____	4. a reddened, swollen, hot, and often painful physical condition
_____	5. of the heart, or pertaining to the heart

   ```
   cardiac
   cholesterol
   fever
   inflammation
   rupture
   surgery
   ```

2. Using Keywords

記事の全体像を理解するために，段落ごとの内容を書き留める習慣をつけておくと効果的です。下記の英文は *Reading* で採り上げた記事中の 7 つの段落の内容を簡潔にまとめたものですが，それぞれが何番目の段落のことなのか，1 〜 7 の番号を付けて示しなさい。

_____ Fatty plaque inside an artery

_____ The role of statins and other drugs in the management of cholesterol

_____ Hormone management of inefficient pumping of the weakened heart

_____ Prevention of heart disease through improved lifestyle

_____ The fight against inflammation

_____ The rationale behind surgery as treatment for heart disease

_____ Genetically related drugs

3. True or False

本文の内容と一致するものに **True**，一致しないものには **False** を記入しなさい。

_____ 1. In spite of the discovery of new drugs, doctors still regard surgery as the best treatment of heart disease.

_____ 2. Doctors are relying more on drugs than before because drugs present fewer risks than surgery.

_____ 3. The human-genome project has contributed greatly to treatment of heart disease.

_____ 4. The reason a fatty deposit becomes inflamed and ruptures has now been clarified.

_____ 5. Drugs called statins are effective on all cardiac patients.

_____ 6. Aspirin can relieve inflammation and make the blood thin.

_____ 7. Congestive heart failure is a disorder related to a fatty deposit inside the coronary artery.

_____ 8. Some hormones exert a significant influence on the heart action.

_____ 9. Even if we exercise vigorously, the risk of suffering heart disease will never lessen.

_____ 10. A healthy lifestyle such as getting enough exercise and keeping a low-calorie diet will reduce the chance of developing heart disease.

4. **Sorting Out the Details**

下の枠から正解を選び，下線部に記入して文を完成させなさい。

This author gives two arguments on why drugs may be better than surgery for treating heart diseases in the future. One reason is that _____

_____

_____

The second reason is that _____

_____

_____

---

people are improving their lifestyles

many smokers are quitting the smoking habit

different kinds of drugs can be prescribed in safe combinations now

the human-genome project will make it possible to individualize each patient's treatment

surgery can remove fatty plaques from the arteries

people at risk of heart disease can now be identified at an early stage of their condition

drugs will play a greater role in the near future

5. Test Yourself on the Gist of this Medical Feature

下記の質問に対する答を英語で書きなさい。

1. Why does the title say "Rethinking"? それぞれの選択肢から1つを選択。

The title says "Rethinking" because doctors are ① _____

② _____ . ③ _____ is

④ _____ ⑤ _____ .

⑥ _____ doctors believe that ⑦ _____ may be able to target

the specific problems and pose fewer risks ⑧ _____ .

① reconsiderate of what	⑤ than previous
reconsidering what	than before times
think again about what	than before

② are the most effective treatments	⑥ This is the reason because
treatments are the most effective	However,
is the cause of heart attacks	As a result,

③ A disease	⑦ surgery
Heart disease	drugs
Its disease	aspirin

④ better understanding today	⑧ than surgery
known more today	than drugs
better understood today	than aspirin

2. What important point is fundamental to our understanding of heart attacks? 選択肢から9つを使って英文で答をつくりなさい。

According to this article, ① _____ ② _____

③ _____ ④ _____ ⑤ _____

⑥ _____ ⑦ _____ ⑧ _____

⑨ _____

| at | attacks | coronary artery damage | heavy drinking of alcohol |
| heart | lies | most | root | of | stress | the |

6. Using What You Know

In **Figure 3.1**, write <u>Left</u> or <u>Right</u> where appropriate, and write <u>Inferior</u> or <u>Superior</u> beside each vena cava.

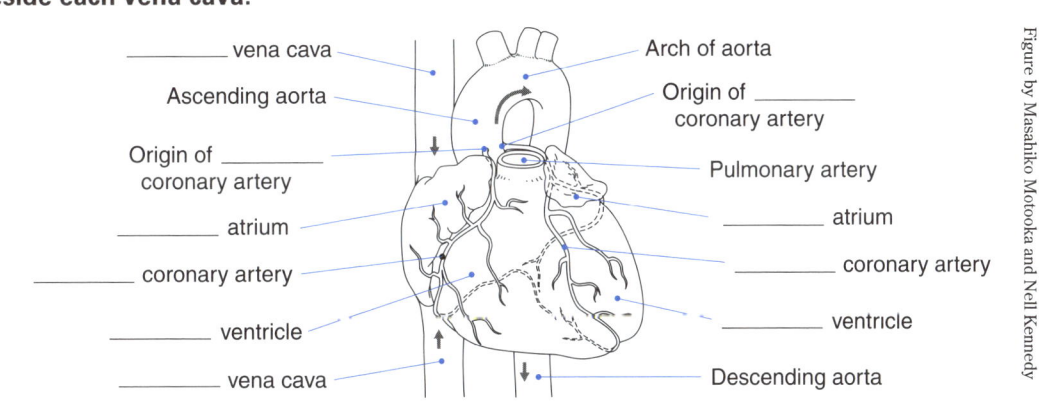

_____ vena cava
Ascending aorta
Origin of _____ coronary artery
_____ atrium
_____ coronary artery
_____ ventricle
_____ vena cava

Arch of aorta
Origin of _____ coronary artery
Pulmonary artery
_____ atrium
_____ coronary artery
_____ ventricle
Descending aorta

Figure by Masahiko Motooka and Nell Kennedy

Figure 3.1. Coronary arteries.

For the text below, choose one answer each and write A–L from the box (some answers are used more than once).

The heart does not take nourishment from the ① _____ that passes through the four chambers inside the heart. Instead, the heart is fed by the left ② _____ and the right ③ _____. The ④ _____ are the first arteries of the body that originate directly from the ⑤ _____, which is the largest artery of the body. Therefore, just after the newly ⑥ _____ blood is pumped out of the ⑦ _____, the coronary arteries and their branches carry the blood-borne nutrients to the ⑧ _____.

A. aorta	B. blood	C. coronary artery	D. coronary arteries
E. deoxygenated	F. heart muscle	G. left	H. left ventricle
I. oxygenated	J. pulmonary artery	K. right	L. right ventricle

7. Crossword Puzzle

下記の定義に従ってマス目を大文字で埋めなさい。

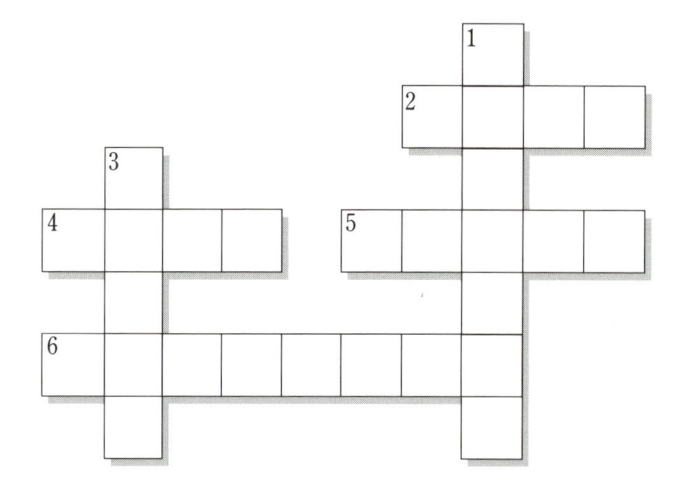

ACROSS

2. exposed to danger, at _____
4. blood vessel carrying blood toward the heart
5. to apply medical care
6. blood vessels carrying blood away from the heart

DOWN

1. illness, an unhealthy condition of the body
3. the organ that pumps blood

Checkpoint　多くの学生が，plaque と書くべきところを誤って plague と書き，また diseased を deceased, heart を hart と書いてしまいます。drugs と drags もよく間違えます。あなたはどうですか？ heartbeat（心拍）は ear で聴きますから，heart の中には ear があると覚えておきましょう。

注意： plaque（斑，プラーク）　　plague（疫病，災害）
　　　 diseased（病気にかかった）　deceased（死去した）
　　　 heart（心臓，心）　　　　　 hart（雄ジカ）
　　　 drug（薬）　　　　　　　　 drag（ひっぱる，ひきずる）

Part 2
Listening to Medical News Reports

Part 2: Listening to Medical News Reports

Chapter 4 Drugs for High Blood Pressure

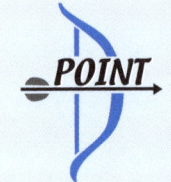

> **POINT**　Chapter 4 では比較的ゆっくりとしたスピードの英語放送を聴きます。最初は内容を大まかに把握し，段階的に細部を理解していきましょう。

Exercises 1, 2 では放送全体を聴き，概要を把握します。Exercises 3 〜 6 では放送の一部を聴き，細かな内容を把握します。Exercise 7 では，もう一度放送全体を聴き，理解した内容を確認します。最後の Exercise 8 では報道内容について元となった論文を参照しながら解説します。

Exercises CD

1. Vocabulary

放送全体を聴き，放送中に実際に使われている重要語句を **1 〜 10** の中から **5** つ選び，その重要語句を和訳しなさい。(**CD tracks 4–8**)

1. the bladder	2. blood vessel	3. costly medicines	4. diuretics
5. drug abuse	6. experiment	7. heart disease	8. high blood pressure
9. stroke	10. urology		

［語句］_____　［和訳］_____

［語句］_____　［和訳］_____

［語句］_____　［和訳］_____

［語句］ _____ ［和訳］ _____

［語句］ _____ ［和訳］ _____

2. Comprehension

放送全体を聴き，次の 1 〜 5 について，話の内容の順に並べなさい。（**CD tracks 4–8**）

1. An institute in Maryland conducted the largest study of high blood pressure ever in the United States.

2. Doctors currently use newer drugs rather than diuretics.

3. Many people around the world have high blood pressure and use diuretics.

4. A new study showed the advantage of one of the diuretics over some of the more expensive drugs with regard to efficacy and cost.

5. Three kinds of medicines were used in the study on high blood pressure.

順序 ☐ → ☐ → ☐ → ☐ → ☐
   1st   2nd   3rd   4th   5th

3. Comprehension

放送の冒頭部分を聴き，次の質問に英語で答えなさい。（**CD track 5**）

1. How many Americans have high blood pressure?

   _____

2. What is the main cause of heart failure and strokes?

   _____

4. **Listening**

冒頭に続く部分を聴き，空欄に語句を埋めなさい。（**CD track 6**）

1. Diuretics _____ high blood pressure _____ than the more expensive drugs did.

2. Diuretics _____ heart failure and strokes _____ _____ than the costly medicines.

3. Diuretics are _____ times cheaper than one of the costly medicines in the study.

5. **Listening**

放送の中盤部分を聴き，次の表を埋めなさい。（**CD track 7**）

研究実施機関の名称	
研究の開始年	
被験者数	
被験者の平均年齢	
使用薬剤	

6. **Comprehension**

放送の終盤を聴き，次の質問に英語で答えなさい。（**CD track 8**）

1. On average, how long did these researchers study the patients' progress?

   _____

2. Which medicines lowered blood pressure?

   _____

3. How long have doctors been using diuretics for their patients?

_____

4. Who approved the more costly drugs?

_____

7. True or False

もう一度放送全体を聴き，次の英文について放送内容と合致するものに **True**，合致しないものに **False** を記入しなさい。(**CD tracks 4–8**)

_____ 1. This study included 50-million Americans.

_____ 2. This research was conducted in one hospital in Bethesda, Maryland.

_____ 3. One of the expensive medicines cost about two dollars for each pill.

_____ 4. The American Medical Association led the study in 1994.

_____ 5. Many more women and blacks participated in the latest study than in earlier studies.

_____ 6. The costly drugs reduced the risk of heart trouble and strokes better than diuretics.

_____ 7. Diuretics have become increasingly popular during the past 20 years.

8. Training to Listen like a Scientist

巻末にある **Appendix**（p. 137）を読み，**VOA** の報道と，その出所となっている研究論文とでは，どのような類似点・相違点があるかを確かめなさい。(**CD track 9**)

Go to page 137

For Further Study　CD

以下の単語の発音を練習しなさい。(CD track 10)

high blood pressure	pill
heart failure	The National Heart, Lung and Blood Institute
stroke	*Journal of the American Medical Association*
heart attack	heart disease
diuretics	calcium channel blocker
sodium	ACE inhibitor (ACE: angiotensin-converting enzyme)
urine	progress
liquid	heart trouble
waste	order
prevent	The United States Food and Drug Administration

Checkpoint　英語のリスニングにおいて重要になってくるのが，単語力です。知っている単語が多い場合には耳に入ってくる情報量が多くなりますが，知らない単語が連続すると理解はかなり困難になります。単語を覚える際には，単語を音と結びつけて覚えることが大切です。ビタミンと英単語の vitamin が綴り字や意味で結びついていても，[váɪtəmɪn]（ヴァイタミン）という音と結びついていなければ，リスニングで理解することはできません。医学英単語を覚えるとき，特にカタカナになっている用語を覚えるときには，必ず音と結びつけるようにしてください。電子辞書や CD−ROM 版の辞書には，音声を聴くことができるものがありますので活用しましょう。

The medical news report in this Chapter is reproduced from "Drugs for High Blood Pressure," VOA Special English / Health Report. January 8, 2003. Copyright ©2003 VOA. Used with permission from voanews.com, Voice of America.

COLUMN

VOA Special English について

　Voice of America（VOA）の Special English は，英語を母国語としない人を対象としたニュース番組です。放送はノーマルスピードの3分の2程度に抑えてあります。頻繁に使用される語彙は1500語程度で，一つ一つのセンテンスが簡潔につくられているために，内容を容易に理解することができます。放送の内容を細かい部分まで理解する練習に最適です。インターネットで放送のスクリプト，音声ファイルを無料で入手することができます。放送を数回聴いてニュースの内容を理解できるようになることを目標に，インターネットに実際にアクセスし，練習を繰り返しましょう。

放送局のインターネットアドレス
〈http://www.voanews.com/specialenglish/〉

　VOA Special English のホームページの下の欄に Topics が並んでいます。Health & Medicine をクリックすると，最近のニュースが順に並んだページが表示されます。ニュースのヘッドラインをクリックすることで，ニュースのスクリプト，音声ファイルが置かれているページが表示されます。過去の放送については，Transcript Archive を開いてください。過去の放送が1週間ずつまとめてあります。このテキストで使用した Health Report は，毎週火曜日に放送されています。

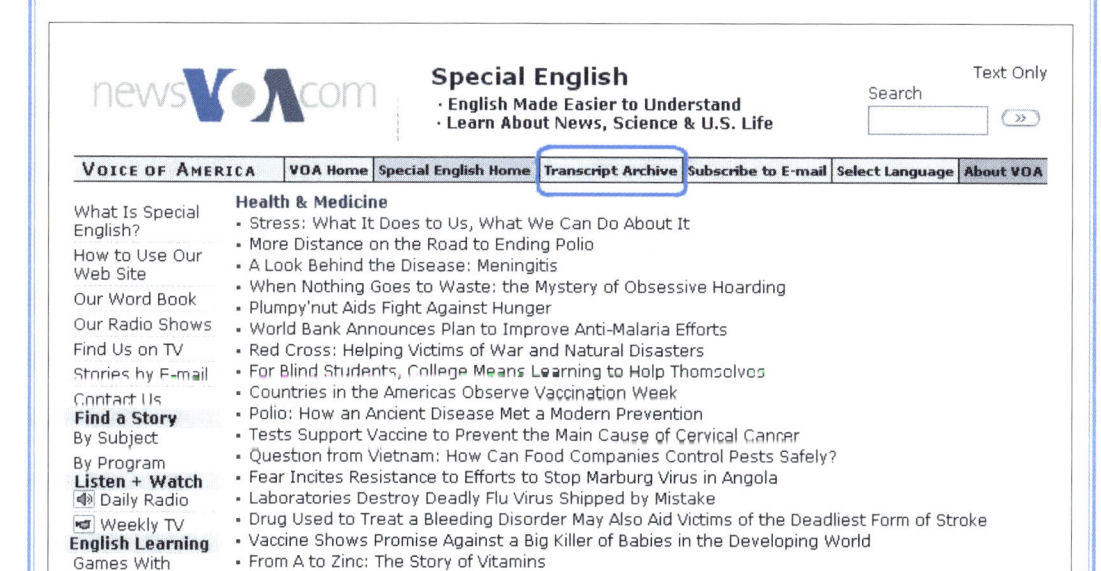

Part 2: Listening to Medical News Reports

Chapter 5 The Battle between HIV and Antibodies

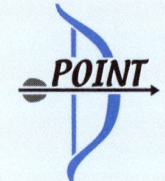

POINT

Chapter 5 ではノーマルスピードの英語放送を聴きます。Chapter 4 と同様に，最初は内容を大まかに把握し，段階的に細部を理解していきましょう。

Exercises CD

1. Vocabulary

放送全体を聴き，放送中に実際に使われている重要語句を 1 ～ 7 の中からそれぞれ 1 つ選び，その重要語句を和訳しなさい。(**CD tracks 11–13**)

1.	AIDS	cancer	heart disease	influenza	obesity
2.	allergy	blood clot	cholesterol	tumor	virus
3.	diet	drip	drug	injection	vaccine
4.	digestion	immune	metabolism	respiration	sympathetic nerve
5.	complication	infection	inflammation	metastasis	remission
6.	blood	lymphocyte	platelet	tissue	white blood cell
7.	incubation	invasion	mutation	proliferation	tolerance

1. ［語句］ _____ ［和訳］ _____

2. ［語句］ _____ ［和訳］ _____

3. ［語句］ _____ ［和訳］ _____

4. ［語句］ _____ ［和訳］ _____

5. ［語句］ _____ ［和訳］ _____

6. ［語句］ _____ ［和訳］ _____

7. ［語句］ _____ ［和訳］ _____

2. Comprehension

放送の冒頭部分を聴き，次の質問に英語で答えなさい。(**CD track 11**)

1. **Fill in each blank with an appropriate verb.**

    a. When the body is infected with a virus, the immune system _____ _____ antibodies.

    b. Antibodies _____ or _____ _____ infection.

    c. The neutralizing antibodies _____ and _____ invading germs.

2. **Which best describes the new finding?**

    a. When the human body is infected with HIV, the immune system controls the infection.

    b. HIV can be eliminated from the body with the neutralizing antibodies.

    c. HIV evolves into new strains before the patient's body can eliminate the virus.

    d. Researchers succeeded in developing a new AIDS vaccine.

    Answer: _____

3. Comprehension

放送の中盤部分を聴き，次の質問に英語で答えなさい。(**CD track 12**)

1. **Who is Dr. Douglas Richman?**

    _____

2. **Dr. Richman says, "It makes mistakes." What does this sentence mean?**

    a. HIV makes errors when replicating the genetic material.

    b. Human beings make mistakes many times a day.

    c. The Darwinian theory of evolution fails to account for the proliferation of the HIV virus.

    d. The antibody cannot recognize the different strains of HIV.

    Answer: _____

3. **In the fight between the antibodies and HIV, six stages are involved. Put them in the right order.**

   a. The antibodies evolve to recognize variations in the virus.

   b. The virus continues to change quickly.

   c. The antibodies begin to attack HIV.

   d. The virus replicates and mutates at an astonishing rate.

   e. The neutralizing antibody response cannot keep up with the changes in the virus.

   f. The mutated form of the virus becomes predominant.

   順序 ☐ → ☐ → ☐ → ☐ → ☐ → f
      1st   2nd   3rd   4th   5th   6th

4. **Comprehension**

   放送の終盤部分を聴き，次の質問に英語で答えなさい。（**CD track 13**）

   1. **Why are scientists taking an optimistic view despite the new findings?**

      a. Because the virus replicates only one hundred billion times.

      b. Because the immune system is one step ahead of HIV.

      c. Because the antibody response might be useful for the prevention of new infections.

      d. Because the antibody turns out to be effective in dealing with an ongoing infection.

      Answer: _____

   2. **According to these researchers, what is necessary for an AIDS vaccine to work?**

      _____

   3. **According to Dr. Richman, how long will it take to develop an effective AIDS vaccine?**

      _____

5. **True or False**

もう一度放送全体を聴き，次の英文について放送内容と合致するものに **True**，合致しないものに **False** を記入しなさい。（**CD tracks 11–13**）

_____ 1. HIV is the virus that causes AIDS.

_____ 2. The study by Dr. Richman showed how HIV stays one step ahead of the antibody response.

_____ 3. Darwinian-like evolution occurs fast and furiously as the result of HIV reproduction.

_____ 4. Prophylaxis is one kind of vaccine to prevent HIV infection.

_____ 5. Dr. Richman criticized the optimistic results raised by the antibody study.

_____ 6. Clinical trials for an AIDS vaccine will be possible in a few years.

For Further Study

以下の単語の発音を練習しなさい。（CD track 14）

HIV	strain	progeny
the immune system	vaccine	Darwinian evolution
antibody	virologist	particle
infection	replicate	selective pressure
neutralizing antibody	mutate	selective force
germ	variation	prophylaxis
antibody response	mutation	
evolve	genetic material	

COLUMN

VOA News について

Voice of America（VOA）は世界のさまざまな地域に向けてニュースを提供しています。VOA English News では，健康を話題にしたニュースがほぼ毎日配信されています。また，アフリカ地域に向けた，VOA English to Africa では，毎週医療情報を提供し，AIDS 問題を特集するなど，医学関連の放送が多数あります。これらのニュースは，ノーマルスピードで放送されているために，最初は聴き取りが難しいと感じるかもしれません。特に，放送の中でインタビューに応じる専門家の英語は，アナウンサーや記者に比べて発音に癖があり，録音状態があまり良くないときもあります。しかし，これがより実践的な英語を聴く良い訓練となります。リスニングが苦手という人のほとんどが聴き取りの練習時間が足りません。最初は，ニュースの内容を理解することよりも，さまざまな人が話す英語の発音やスピードに慣れることを目標にして，ニュースを大量に，そして集中して聴いてください。「英語耳」をつくるために「まずは 100 時間を目標に！」とも言われています。

放送局のインターネットアドレス
VOA English News:
〈http://www.voanews.com/english/〉
VOA English to Africa:
〈http://www.voanews.com/english/africa/〉

放送のスクリプトと音声ファイルを無料で入手することができます。VOA English News のホームページにある Topic の中から，あるいは Site Map の News Categories の中から，Health を選択することで，健康関連のページに入ることができます。また，VOA English to Africa のホームページには，AIDS の特集，医療情報の特集のバナーを選択することで，ニュースやレポートの一覧を見ることができます。過去の放送を視聴するためには，Search VOA から検索をしましょう。キーワードを入力することで，類似する内容の放送を多数聴くことができます。

newsVOA.com

A trusted source of news and information since 1942

Text Only
Search

VOICE OF AMERICA | VOA Home | VOA English | Regions/Topics | Subscribe to E-mail | Select Language | About VOA

Stories by Topic (most recent at the top)

LISTEN TO VOA
Latest Newscast
News Now Live

PROGRAMS A TO Z
Find VOA Radio or TV Programs
Webcasts
Audience Mail
Correspondents

REGIONS
Africa
Americas
Asia
Europe
Middle East
U.S.A.

VOA IN-DEPTH
American Life
Health & Science
Entertainment
News Analysis

LEARNING ENGLISH
Articles in *Special English*

EDITORIALS
Read Editorials

Health
- President Clinton to Undergo More Surgery Thursday
- Study: Fetuses of Pregnant Smokers at Higher Risk of Genetic Mutations Linked to Leukemia
- Women in Ivory Coast Fight HIV-AIDS Stigma
- Public Health Experts Draw Attention to Saving Newborn Babies in Developing World
- Scientists Examine Protein's Possible Connection to Longevity
- UN: Hazardous Waste Dumped on Somali Shores by Tsunami
- Pope to Make Silent Blessing From Hospital Window Sunday
- HIV/AIDS: Three Scenarios For Africa
- UNAIDS Lays Out Scenarios From Dire to Hopeful for Africa
- UN Sees Up to 83 Million AIDS Deaths in Africa by 2025
- Experts: Simple Measures Can Avert Millions of Infant Deaths a Year
- World Faces Major Challenges in AIDS Battle, US Says
- UN: Drug Trafficking and Abuse On the Rise in Africa
- Global Fund Cuts Off Malaria Grant for Senegal
- Afghan Feminist Urges Nations to Invest in Women as Emerging Leaders Who Can Transform Their Communities
- UN Report Warns of Rise in Heroin Abuse, Spread of AIDS
- Modern Dental Problems Blamed on Advent of Cooking
- Polio Vaccination Campaign Under Way Across Africa
- Activists Urge Hollywood to Cut Back on Smoking in Movies
- UN: Polio Spreading from Sudan

FAQs | Terms of Use & Privacy Notice | Broadcasting Board of Governors | Site Map | Contact Us

---

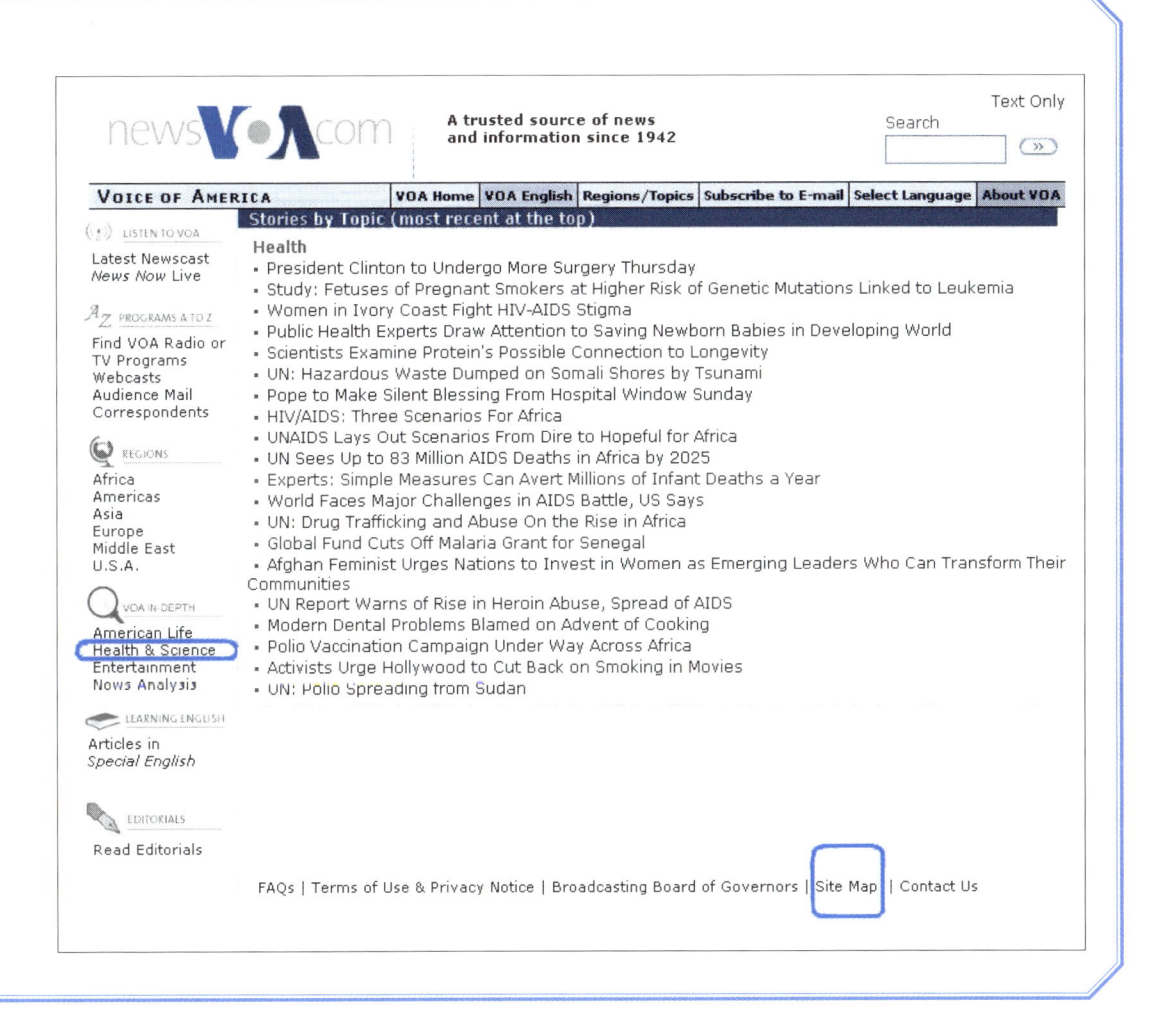

The medical news report in this Chapter is reproduced from "The Battle between HIV and Antibodies: Why the Virus Gets the Upper Hand," VOA English for Africa. March 20, 2003. Copyright ©2003 VOA. Used with permission from voanews.com, Voice of America.

Part 2: Listening to Medical News Reports

Chapter 6 Drug to Stop Progression of Type 1 Diabetes

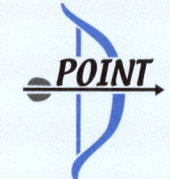

POINT Chapter 6 では，Chapter 5 と同様に，ノーマルスピードの英語放送を聴きます。

Exercises CD

1. Vocabulary

女性キャスターに続いて，3 人の男性が登場します。放送に出てくる順番に「氏名」を書いた上で，それぞれの「身分」，「所属」について語群から選び，表を埋めなさい。（**CD tracks 15–20**）

登場順	氏名	身分	所属
1.	_____	_____	_____
2.	_____	_____	_____
3.	_____	_____	_____

氏名	Kevan C. Herold	Richard Harris	Robert Goldstein
身分	Chief science officer	News reporter	University researcher
所属	Columbia University The Juvenile Diabetes Research Foundation	NPR Washington	UC San Francisco

注：Dr. Kevan C. Herold は一流の医学誌に数多くの論文が掲載されている研究者ですが，NPR が配信するスクリプトでは Dr. Kevin "Harold" と記され，綴りが誤っています。Harold は通常，名（first name）として用いられますが，姓（family name）としては用いられません。本書ではご本人に確認したうえで，正しい綴りで表記しています。

2. **Vocabulary**

放送全体を聴き，放送中に実際に使われている重要語句を 1 〜12 の中から 6 つ選び，その重要語句を和訳しなさい。（**CD tracks 15–20**）

1. antibody
2. complication
3. fat
4. glucose
5. immune
6. insulin
7. juvenile diabetes
8. lifestyle
9. the liver
10. nephropathy
11. the pancreas
12. side effect

[語句] _____ [和訳] _____

[語句] _____ [和訳] _____

[語句] _____ [和訳] _____

[語句] _____ [和訳] _____

[語句] _____ [和訳] _____

[語句] _____ [和訳] _____

3. **Comprehension**

放送の前半部分では，レポーターと博士が交互に話をしています。それぞれ，どのようなことをテーマに話をしているか，1 〜 5 の中から選び，下線部に番号を入れなさい。同じテーマで話しているときには，記号を繰り返し用いることができます。（**CD track 16**）

Reporter: _____

Doctor: _____

Reporter: _____

Doctor: _____

Reporter: _____

Doctor: _____

Reporter: _____

1. An outline of the new treatment.
2. A short description of type 1 diabetes.
3. Conventional therapy and its side effects.
4. Possible long-term effects of this new treatment.
5. The results of the treatment.

注： Diabetes の type の表記に関しては一部でローマ数字も用いられていますが, the American Diabetes Association 等の専門機関では，"type 1(2) diabetes" のようにアラビア数字を使用しています。

4. Listening

前半の一部分を聴き，空欄に語句を埋めなさい。（**CD track 16**）

Insulin is produced by ① _____ _____ , and it controls

② _____ _____ . Type 1 diabetes, which used to be called

③ _____ diabetes, is a disease of ④ _____ _____

_____ .

5. Comprehension

前半の一部分を聴き，質問に答えなさい。（**CD track 17**）

According to this report, which statement about immune suppressive drugs is <u>NOT</u> correct?

   a. The immune suppressive drugs are effective in short-term studies.

   b. Several kinds of immune suppressive drugs should be used for short periods each.

   c. The immune suppressive drugs have been shown to cause serious side effects.

   d. The risks of infection and tumors increase if the immune suppressive drugs are used for a long period.

   Answer: _____

6. Listening

前半の一部分を聴き，空欄に語句を埋めなさい。（**CD track 18**）

In this study, a ① _____ _____ _____ was tested in

human beings for the first time. ② _____ subjects participated in the test

for ③ _____ _____ . The side effects of the treatment were

④ _____ .

7. Comprehension

前半の一部分を聴き，質問に答えなさい。（**CD track 19**）

What is the main benefit of the antibody-based drug treatment?

    a. The patients retain their ability to make insulin.

    b. About 49% of the patients have no side effects.

    c. The patients no longer need insulin injections.

    d. Even a modest dose of the new drug is more effective than a full dose of conventional drugs.

    Answer: _____

8. True or False

放送の後半部分を聴き，次の英文について放送内容と合致するものに **True**，合致しないものに **False** を記入しなさい。（**CD track 20**）

_____ 1. Dr. Goldstein thinks it is too early to evaluate the success of the new treatment.

_____ 2. Dr. Goldstein thinks the therapeutic effect of the new treatment and long-term effects of the new treatment must be studied further to confirm the safety and efficacy of the drug for clinical use.

_____ 3. Dr. Goldstein expects harmful effects on the immune system when the new treatment is used for a long period.

_____ 4. Similar experiments using antibody-based drugs have not shown satisfactory results.

_____ 5. Dr. Goldstein is also looking for applications of antibody-based drugs to diseases besides diabetes.

_____ 6. Dr. Goldstein wants to know whether the antibody-based treatment is useful for the prevention of diabetes.

_____ 7. Dr. Goldstein has already expanded the study by Dr. Herold to include more volunteers.

_____ 8. Mr. Harris concluded his report with a pessimistic view of the prospects of the new drug.

For Further Study CD

以下の単語の発音を練習しなさい。(CD track 21)

type 1 diabetes	chronic
The New England Journal of Medicine	antibody
the pancreas	diabetics
insulin	genetically engineered
blood sugar	diagnose
juvenile diabetes	injection
the immune system	modest
immune response	shot
immune suppressive drug	chief scientific officer
cyclosporine	Juvenile Diabetes Research Foundation
azathioprine	preliminary
prednisone	insulin-secreting cell
kidney disease	collaborator
infection	dose
tumor	

The medical news report in this Chapter is reproduced from "All Things Considered / Type 1 Diabetes," National Public Radio. May 29, 2002. Copyright ©2002 NPR, Inc. Used with permission from National Public Radio, Inc.

COLUMN

NPR について

　National Public Radio（NPR）は，アメリカの国民向けの公共ラジオ放送局です。インターネットを通じて聴くことができるニュース音声ファイル数は世界有数です。ニュース，討論，インタビューなど，多種多様なプログラムが提供されています。

放送局のインターネットアドレス
〈http://www.npr.org〉

　ホームページの左のコラムに，テーマ別のページ，プログラムのページなどへのリンクがあります。Health & Science からは，健康に関する話題を集めたページに入ることができます。Morning Edition という番組は，毎日，ニュースや話題となっていることを手短にまとめています。All Things Considered という番組は，専門家を招いて，時事的な話題を掘り下げています。この章はこの番組で放送されたものを収めています。その他にもさまざまなプログラムが用意されていますが，過去に放送されたニュースはキーワード検索することで，遡って聴くことができます。各ニュースのテキストは，放送の概要を述べたものだけで，スクリプトを入手する場合には有料となります。VOA で実力をつけたら，NPR にチャレンジしてください。

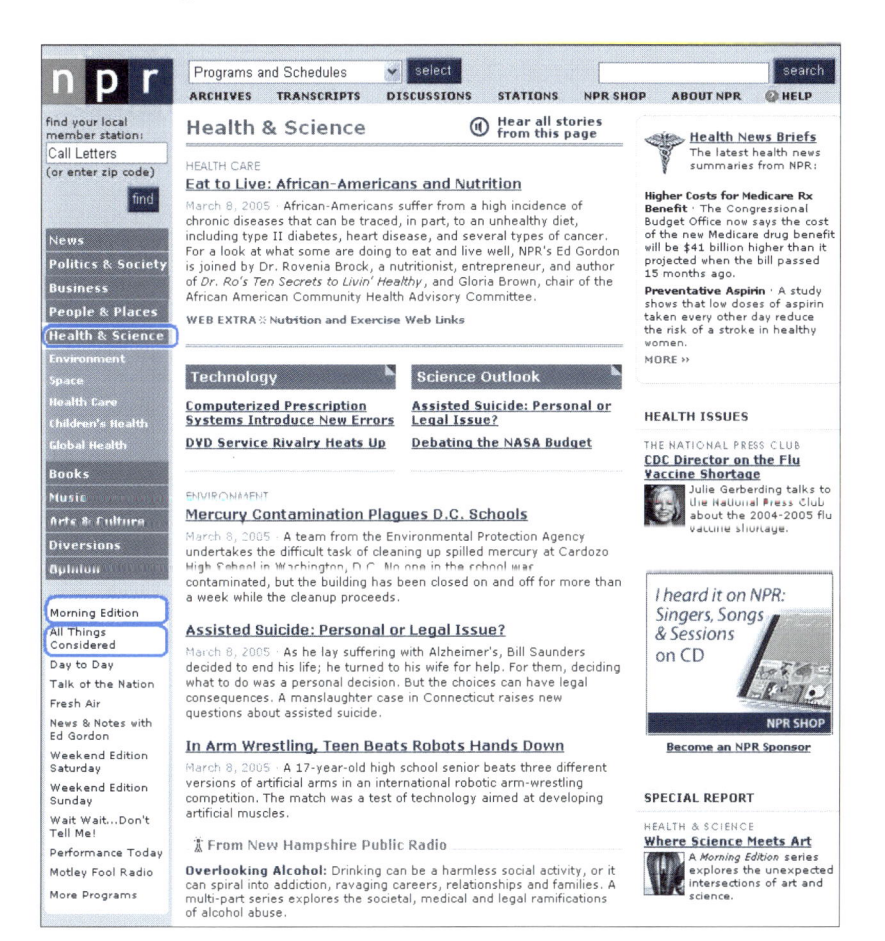

お薦めのリスニング・インターネット無料サイト

■ラジオ放送局

(1) NHK WORLD ラジオ日本 〈http://www.nhk.or.jp/rj/〉

　日本のニュースが英語を含めた 22 の言語で放送されています。日本語でも放送されていますから，内容を常に確認することができます。理解した内容については，英語も聴き取りが簡単です。本書で紹介した英語放送が難しいと感じた人は，ここからスタートするのもよいでしょう。また，身近な話題を英語で話すための訓練として，日常的に聴いて語彙力を蓄えるのも一つの利用方法です。

(2) The World 〈http://www.theworld.org/〉

　BBC を初め，いくつかの放送局で流されたニュースを集めたサイトです。音声ファイルをダウンロードすることができますので，パソコン，携帯プレーヤーなどにダウンロードして，リスニングの練習をすることができます。スクリプトは一切提供されていません。

(3) BBC 〈http://www.bbc.co.uk/radio/〉

　本書で取り上げた放送局はすべてアメリカに本局をおいていますが，BBC はイギリスの国営放送局です。インターネットで配信している音声ファイルとスクリプトは世界最大規模です。特に，BBC Radio 4 の Science (http://www.bbc.co.uk/radio4/science/) では，医学に関してもかなり専門的な内容を扱っています。ニュースでは物足りない人はぜひチャレンジしてみてください。

■テレビ放送局

(1) CBS News 〈http://www.cbsnews.com/〉

　Free CBS News Video のページを開くと，ニュース番組を視聴することができます。左のコラムに Health があるので，健康関連の話題に絞ることができます。映像の助けがあるので，多少聴き取れない部分があっても全体の内容は理解することができます。

(2) Healthology 〈http://www.healthology.com〉

　医学の専門的な内容を放送するサイトです。専門家が多数登場して，さまざまな疾患について解説していきます。クリップも多数出てきますので，視覚的に内容が理解できるようになっています。放送のスクリプト，また内容に関するクイズが用意されている放送もあります。超お薦めサイトです。

Part 3
Reading the Medical Research Paper

Part 3: Reading the Medical Research Paper

Chapter 7　Entering the Medical Research Paper

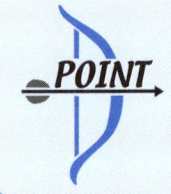

POINT
- 探すべき情報は何か。
- 探している情報がどこにあるか。

Lecture

医学論文入門

　医学論文とは主として医師のために書かれたもので，医学会の雑誌に載っています。最新の確固とした証拠（evidence）に照らし合わせて，いろいろな論文が書かれます。古い技術に異論を唱える論文，よりよい診断，新しくみつかった疾患，ある治療法に対する警告の論文等々です。一般の読者を対象にした medical features や news reports とは内容，構成，目的の点で大きく異なります。ですから医学論文を初めて読む人にとっては，その読み方も目新しいものに感じられると思います。医学論文はかなり専門的なものですし，5〜20ページ程度の分量がありますので，一語一語読んでいくのは上手な読み方とはいえません。

　しかし，ありがたいことにどの医学論文でも主なセクションは4つしかありません。それぞれのセクションには特徴があり，相互に密に関連しています。医学生なら誰でも論文を読む技術を身につけられるでしょう。初めが肝心です。適切な読み方を身につけることが大変重要です。

see p. 62, The Research Problem

see p. 105, Figure 10.1

Title

論文のタイトルには，以下に示してあるような重要な問いの答えが2つ，時には3つ書いてあるはずです。

1. **What <u>topic</u> is the paper about?**
   - ☐ What disease?   ☐ What risk?
   - ☐ What technique?   ☐ What comparison?
   - ☐ What old theory re-examined?   ☐ What trial?

2. **Is the paper based on <u>clinical</u> research or is it based on <u>animal</u> experiments?**
   - ☐ タイトルに healthy volunteers, children with diabetes, pregnant women with HIV のような subgroup があれば，その論文は <u>clinical research</u> についてのものだと考えられます。
   - ☐ タイトルに実験動物の種の記載があれば，その論文は間違いなく <u>experimental research</u> についてのものです。
   - ☐ もし人の subgroup も動物の種もタイトルに書かれてなければ，その論文はたぶん clinical research だと考えられます。

   pregnant: 妊娠している

3. **What is the research focus, or angle?**
   - ☐ Prevention?
   - ☐ Diagnosis?
   - ☐ Treatment?
   - ☐ Basic research?
     - (i) Pathophysiology
     - (ii) Mechanism
     - (iii) Function

   prevention: 予防
   diagnosis: 診断
   treatment: 治療
   basic research: 基礎研究
   pathophysiology: 病態生理学

Exercises

1. Finding vital information in the Title

From each title below, write the <u>topic</u> of the research and whether the research is <u>experimental</u> or <u>clinical</u>. In the titles, underline the key words that tell the disease.

1. Major outcomes in high-risk <u>hypertensive</u> patients randomized to angiotensin-converting enzyme inhibitor or calcium channel blocker vs diuretic

   research topic   research category

   __hypertension__   __clinical__

   1. Original paper from which the medical news report was compiled, Chapter 4

   inhibitor: 阻害因子，阻害薬
   vs (= versus): 〜対〜

2. Anti-CD3 monoclonal antibody in new-onset type 1 diabetes mellitus

   research topic   research category

   _____   _____

   2. Original paper from which the medical news report was compiled, Chapter 6

   type 1 diabetes: insulin-dependent diabetes

3. Diagnosis of migraine in children at a pediatric headache clinic

   research topic   research category

   _____   _____

   pediatric: 小児〔科〕の

4. The effect of oral sucrose on exercise tolerance in patients with McArdle's disease

   research topic   research category

   _____   _____

   exercise tolerance: 運動耐容能

5. Role of mitochondrial nitric oxide in rat heart and kidney during hypertension

   research topic   research category

   _____   _____

   nitric oxide (NO): 一酸化窒素

6. Preventive effects of a soy-based diet on the development of type 2 diabetes in Zucker diabetic fatty rats

research topic

research category

_____   _____

Zucker diabetic fatty rat: インスリン非依存性糖尿病（non-insulin-dependent diabetes）のモデル動物

type 2 diabetes: non-insulin-dependent diabetes

2. **Guessing at the research focus in the Title**

On the following lines numbered according to the Titles in Exercise 1 above, write one research focus each: **prevention**, **diagnosis**, **treatment**, or **basic research**.

the research focus   the research focus

1. _____   2. ___treatment_____

3. _____   4. _____

5. _____   6. _____

Lecture

What the Abstract can and cannot do
抄録の役割

　論文のタイトルだけでは必要な情報が十分にわからない場合は，通常，抄録から必要な情報が得られます。

　抄録には subheads が付いているものと付いていないものがありますが，いずれも論文の内容とまったく同じ順に，短くはあってもしっかりと組み立てられて書かれています。

Reading warm-up

The Effect of Oral Sucrose on Exercise Tolerance in Patients with McArdle's Disease

■ Abstract

BACKGROUND. Energy metabolism in muscles relies predominantly on the breakdown of glycogen early in exercise. In patients with McArdle's disease, blocked glycogenolysis in muscles results in low exercise tolerance and can lead to muscle injury, particularly in the first minutes of exercise. We hypothesized that ingesting sucrose before exercise would increase the availability of glucose and would therefore improve exercise tolerance in patients with McArdle's disease.

METHODS. —

RESULTS. —

CONCLUSION. This study suggests that the ingestion of sucrose before exercise can markedly improve exercise tolerance in patients with McArdle's disease.

* Vissing, John and Haller, Ronald G. 2003. The effect of oral sucrose on exercise tolerance in patients with McArdle's disease. *N Eng J Med* **349** (26): 2503–2509. Copyright ©2003 Massachusetts Medical Society. All rights reserved. Translated with permission Nov. 2005. RY–2006–1748.

McArdle's disease: known also as glycogen storage disease type V, and as muscle glycogen phosphorylase deficiency

metabolism: 代謝

predominantly: 主に，だいたいは

glycogenolysis: グリコーゲン（糖原）分解

exercise tolerance: 運動耐容能

sucrose: ショ糖

ingest: 摂取する

hypothesize: 仮説を立てる

Methods, Results: see Chapter 9

■ Underline key words
■ Number the points from the known to the unknown

　医学論文を読むときは，この2点が大変役に立ちます。まずはキーワードを見つけて下線を引くこと，次に著者の論点に番号を振っておくことです。例えばこの抄録の例では，読み慣れた人ならおそらく <u>energy metabolism</u>, <u>glycogen</u>, <u>early in exercise</u>, <u>McArdle's disease</u>, <u>low exercise tolerance</u>, <u>muscle injury</u>, <u>sucrose</u>, <u>glucose</u> というキーワードに下線を引くでしょう。そして，著者の論点はまず現時点でわかっていること，そして未知のこと，最後にこの研究で解明したことへと進みます。

医学論文: a medical research paper

読み慣れた人: seasoned readers

Exercises

3. Understanding the Abstract

1. **Did the results of this study support the authors' hypothesis?**

   Circle A, B, C, or D to show the correct answer.

   A. No, because patients with McArdle's disease cannot metabolize the sugar.

   B. Yes. If the patients ingested sucrose before exercise, they could tolerate the exercise better.

   C. Yes. If the patients ingested sucrose immediately after exercise, they could prevent muscle injury.

   D. We can't answer this question yet because this Abstract does not tell the results of the experiments.

2. **In Exercise 2 (p. 57), we may not be able to figure out whether Title 4 focuses on treatment or on prevention. After reading the Abstract (p. 58), circle the answer you think best (A–D below).**

   A. The research focuses on prevention of McArdle's disease.

   B. The research focuses on treatment, because although sucrose does not prevent McArdle's disease it helps reduce the symptoms.

   C. The research focuses on the treatment of muscle injury after exercise.

   D. The focus of this research is neither on prevention nor on treatment.

4. Composition

Write your answer on the lines.

When we describe a patient in English, the name of the disease usually comes after the word patient. To say 「マッカードル病患者」 in English, we say:

_____ _____ _____ _____

5. Asking questions

In the following case, what questions would a doctor want to answer by reading the research paper that goes with the Title and Abstract on p. 58?

Imagine that a 24-year-old man from Canada presented at your hospital with pain and stiffness in his legs. Six years ago, a doctor diagnosed McArdle's disease in this patient, but no cure is available yet. Last weekend the man helped some friends move a heavy sofa, a filing cabinet, and a few stacks of books. After that, he had to stay in bed for two-and-a-half days because of severe muscle cramps, pain, and fatigue. He came to your clinic because he knows you are a doctor who wants to do evidence-based medicine（科学的根拠に基づく医療，EBM）. After reading this Abstract, you would like to advise this patient to take sucrose the next time he plans to do heavy work or exercise. But the Abstract does not tell enough details.

With classmates, discuss the possibility of sucrose, and list what details you would need to look for inside the main body of the paper. Use expressions such as <u>how much</u>, <u>how long</u>, <u>how soon</u>, <u>what kind</u>.

a. _____

b. _____

c. _____

d. _____

e. _____

Checkpoint 人名が付いている病名（eponyms）には Down's syndrome や Down syndrome のように ['s] が付いている形と付いていない形があります（*Council of Biology Editors Style Manual*）。マッカードル病に関しては，現在ほとんどの雑誌で ['s] が付いている方を使っています。しかし，*the American Medical Association Manual of Style: a guide for authors and editors* はすべて ['s] が付いていない形を使うことを勧めているため，現段階では，雑誌によって付けなくなったり，まだ付いていたりします。人名が付いている疾患に関する論文を書く場合は，投稿する雑誌の様式に従ってください。

Lecture

Pre-reading 準備体操

　運動選手やダンサーは大きな大会の前はもちろん，通常の練習の前にも必ず準備体操や身体のストレッチをします。よい成績をあげるためには欠かせないものです。同様に，医学論文を読むときも論文の本文を読む前に，ある特定の部分を事前に必ず読んでおくと，理解しやすくなり時間も短縮できて楽しく読めます。

　また，特定の部分を読んでおくことで全体がすばやく把握できます。医学論文では概観，つまり全体を掴むことが大変役に立ちます。論文の構成がほとんど同じだからです。ある論文で必要な情報がどこに書いてあるか場所を特定できるようになれば，他のどの論文でも同様の情報を探すのがずっと容易になります。

Entering the Main Body of the Paper

　医学論文を読み始めるにあたって，まず３つの質問を自身に問いかけてみましょう。そうすることによって読む時間がぐんと短縮でき，理解も深まります。

　Q1.　**What** is this paper about?
　Q2.　What is the research **question**, or medical problem?
　Q3.　What is the author's **answer** to the research question?

　次頁の Figure 7.1 で，論文のどこにそれら３つの質問の答えが書かれているかが示してあります。

Q1. Usually found in the first or first two sentences of the Introduction.
Q2. Usually at or near the end of the Introduction.
Q3. Usually in the last paragraph of the Discussion, known as the conclusion. Also commonly found in the opening sentence of the Discussion.

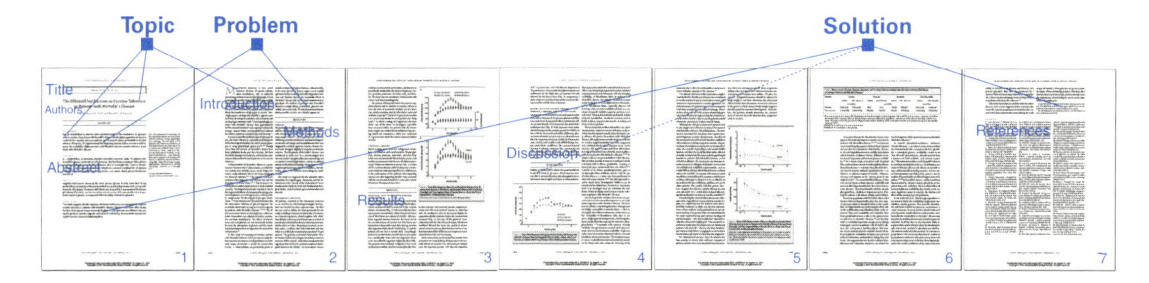

Figure 7.1. Where to start reading the medical research paper.
医学論文をどこから読みはじめるか。この図は，*The New England Journal of Medicine* に掲載されていた7ページの論文での例です。

The Research Problem

　どの科学論文でも research problem，すなわち研究課題が一番の素です。研究課題がなければ，論文の存在意義はありません。医学論文はいずれもある1つの疑問に関することを4つのセクションで語っています。その4つとは，Introduction, Methods, Results, Discussion（IMRD）で，読むときはRとDの間にandを入れてIMRaDと発音しています。4つのセクションはそれぞれ異なる角度から語っていますが，どのセクションも同じ疑問に焦点を当てています（Table 7–1）。

Table 7–1. 医学論文での4つの主なセクションの相互依存関係

IMRD Sections of the Paper	それぞれのセクションが1つの研究課題にどのように焦点をあてているか
Introduction	● 論文の疑問を提示（研究目的） ● それまでの研究でその疑問に対してどのような展開があったか ● この疑問の答えを見つけることの意義
Methods	● この疑問に答えるために何をしたかを詳細に説明
Results	● 研究で得られた結果のデータを提示
Discussion	● データを解釈し，疑問に答える ● 今回得られた答えが，これまでの研究とどのように適合するか，しないのかを述べる ● この答えが世界的に重要である理由を示唆

Chapter 7 Entering the Medical Research Paper

Exercises

6. **Pre-reading 2 spots in the Introduction**

   A. Skip to the <u>first</u> sentence in the Introduction in Chapter 8 (p. 68, line 1), then bring back the answer to Q1 and write your answer on the line below.

   Go to the Introduction (Chapter 8)

   Q1. What is the general topic of this paper? (What is this paper about?)

   This paper is about _____ .

   oral sucrose   exercise tolerance   patients   McArdle's disease

   B. Skip to the <u>last paragraph</u> of the Introduction (lines 45–48) and complete the answer to Q2.

   Q2. What specific question, or problem, were the authors trying to solve?

   (a) The authors were trying to find out _____ patients _____ McArdle's _____ who _____ sucrose _____ before exercise _____ _____ work performance in the early stages of exercise.

   Restate this problem as a question in your own words:

   (b) In patients _____ McArdle's _____ , can _____ sucrose _____ before exercise _____ work performance in the early stages of exercise?

   Restate this problem as a question in your own words:

   (c) If patients _____ McArdle's _____ _____ sucrose orally before exercise, can they _____ their work performance in the early stages of exercise?

63

7. Pre-reading the Conclusion

この問題は研究を終えた後にしか答えられないものなので，論文の最後に近いところまで数ページ跳んで Discussion のセクション（pp. 94–97）を覗いてから戻ってきて，この問題に答えなさい。

Go to the Discussion (Chapter 10)

Q3. What solution, or answer, did the authors find?

(a) The authors _____ that, in _____ _____ McArdle's

_____ , _____ sucrose _____

_____ exercise _____ the _____

_____ and _____ the second-wind phenomenon that

occurs during the early stages of exercise, when the _____ are

_____ _____ muscle injury.

Restate your answer:

(b) This study _____ that the _____ of _____

before _____ can improve exercise _____ in _____

with McArdle's _____ .

Checkpoint 　現在形で記されていると，この研究結果が今回の研究だけでなく一般化することができる，という印になります。

　Conclusion はこの論文のように Discussion セクションの最後のパラグラフに書かれていることがほとんどですが，ジャーナルによっては Discussion セクションの後に改めて Conclusion というセクションを設けてあるものもあります。

For Further Study

Finding other papers and books for doctors

マッカードル病についての医学論文を探すときは，Medline で glycogen storage disease type V あるいは muscle glycogen phosphorylase deficiency といったキーワードで検索します。

文献名の長いリストでは，最初はどれが本のタイトルで，どれが学術誌に掲載された論文なのかわかりにくいものです。下記に判別の手がかりが示してあります。

Medline：米国立医学図書館によるオンライン医学文献検索サービスの名称。

First author's family name / **First name** / **Year of publication**

Kazemi-Esfarjani P, Skomorowska B, Jensen TD, Haller RG, Vissing J. 2002. A nonischemic forearm exercise test for McArdle disease. *Ann Neurol* 52: 153–159.

Page numbers / **Title of the paper** / **Journal** (*Ann Neurol: Annals of Neurology*) / **Volume No.**

First author's family name / **Year of publication** / **Chapter title** / **The book editor**

Vissing J, Haller RG. 2001. Metabolic myopathies. In: Pourmand R, ed. *Neuromuscular Diseases: Expert Clinicians' Views.* Boston: Butterworth–Heinemann, pp. 393–410.

Book title / **Page numbers for this chapter** / **City of publication** / **The book publisher**

Using the Internet to contact patients with McArdle's disease

下記は 24 歳の青年やその他のマッカードル病患者が自分の経験について述べているホームページの URL です。

< http://www.mdausa.org/publications/Quest/q66metabolic.html >

< http://www.mdusa.org/disease.mpd.cfm >

< http://members.aol.com/itsgumby/people.html68 >

A 24-year-old man and other patients with McArdle's disease tell their experiences.

URL: Uniform Resource Locator

COLUMN

Informal Messages from Patients with McArdle's Disease

- One of the main problems we face is obtaining accurate information about this disease.

  この問題で重要なことは，マッカードル病に関して正しい知識を得ることです。

- When I was in elementary school, I was always the last one to come back if we had to run up the hill and back. But I didn't find out until I was almost 30 that there was this disease called McArdle's disease and that I had it.

  小学生の頃，丘を走って登り，下りてくるというとき，いつもビリでした。30歳近くになって，マッカードル病という病気のせいだったということがやっとわかりました。

- Every time we stood on our tiptoes in gym class, I had to be absent a couple of days to get over the stiffness and pain in my legs. But my parents and I had never heard of McArdle's disease, and the gym teacher and coach figured I was just a sissy. So their theory was to toughen me up by making me run extra laps around the track. After that, of course, I had to skip school for days because my muscles were so stiff and painful.

  体育の授業で爪先立ちをするたびに，脚の凝りや痛みが治るまで2日は休まなければなりませんでした。親も私もマッカードル病なんて聞いたことがありませんでしたし，体育の先生やコーチも私のことを弱虫だと思っていました。それでもっと強くしなければと，トラックをさらにもう何周か走らせました。その後は筋肉が固まり，痛くて何日か学校を休まなければならなかったのは言うまでもありません。

■ In an interview with Quest, the online magazine of the Muscular Dystrophy Association of the United States, another person said: <u>My 22-year-old son was diagnosed with McArdle's disease 10 years ago. I am worried about his kidneys</u>, as I never know when he will overuse his muscles and get the dark-colored urine again. Have any advancements been made in the Australian study on gene therapy?
< http://www.mdausa.org/experts/question.cfm?id=2067 >

- Pulling and lifting heavy things can hurt us the most. But <u>I am 24 years old, and I look perfectly normal on the outside</u>. So when people ask me to help them do something like move a big table or push a heavy filing cabinet across the room, I have to say no. Then everybody just looks at me like they think I'm lazy.

  マッカードル病の私たちにとって重いものを引いたり，持ち上げたりするのは一番大変です。<u>私は24歳，外見はまったく普通</u>です。ですから大きなテーブルを動かしたり，中身のいっぱい詰まった重いキャビネットを押したりするときなどに手伝ってほしいと言われるのですが，できない，と答えざるを得ません。みんな私を怠け者というふうに見ます。

- My sister also has McArdle's. Our doctor told us that if we didn't stop all exercise, <u>the muscle damage could lead to kidney failure</u>. But recently I started riding a bicycle just a few minutes a day and also walking. If I start out slowly, it seems to be ok, and I feel a lot better than when I stopped completely.

  私の姉妹もマッカードル病でした。医者は運動をすべて止めなければ<u>筋肉の損傷が腎不全を招く</u>と言いました。でも最近，1日に数分間だけ自転車に乗ったり歩いたりし始めました。ゆっくり始めれば大丈夫ですし，まったく運動をしないよりずっとよさそうです。

Reprinted with permission of the Muscular Dystrophy Association of the United States. All rights reserved. www.mdausa.org

■ To see two color slides explaining what happens inside the muscle cells of patients with McArdle's disease; a high school cheerleader's photo and story; and an interview with Dr. Haller, co-author of the research paper we are reading, go to these websites:

< http://www.mdausa.org/publications/Quest/q114mcardle.cfm >

< http://www.mdausa.org/publications/Quest/q66metabolic3.html >

Part 3: Reading the Medical Research Paper

Chapter 8 Reading the Introduction

The Effect of Oral Sucrose on Exercise Tolerance in Patients with McArdle's Disease

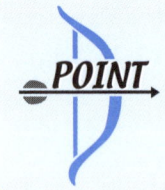

> **POINT**
> - Introduction では，研究を行う前にその研究の正当性を述べます。
> - マッカードル病に関して，未知の重要な医学的知識を探しなさい。
> - 著者が立てる仮説や研究目的は，その未知の部分から発しています。

Reading

CD track 22

Introduction

Q1 McArdle's disease is the most common disorder of muscle carbohydrate metabolism, with an estimated prevalence of about 1 case in 100,000 people. It is an autosomal recessive error of metabolism caused by
5 mutations in the gene that codes for myophosphorylase.[1] Typically, these mutations result in the translation of a nonfunctioning enzyme and completely block the breakdown of glycogen in muscle. Muscle glycogen is an important fuel that supports nearly all muscle
10 energy metabolism early in exercise and during high-intensity work.[2] Correspondingly, patients with McArdle's disease have approximately half the normal maximal work capacity,[3] and muscle cramps, muscle injury, and myoglobinuria induced by sudden, vigorous

disorder: 疾患

metabolism: 代謝

prevalence: 有病率

autosomal recessive error: 常染色体劣性異常

myophosphorylase: 筋ホスホリラーゼ [màɪəfɑsfɔ(ː)rəlèɪs]

enzyme: 酵素

glycogen: グリコーゲン [glάɪkədʒən]

cramps: 痙攣

myoglobinuria: ミオグロビン尿症 [màɪəglòʊbən(j)ʊ́(ə)rɪə]

exercise frequently develop.[4,5]

Because it specifically blocks muscle glycogenolysis, McArdle's disease is a naturally occurring model that has helped elucidate the role of muscle glycogen in many physiologic processes.[3,6–12] Though more than 200 articles on McArdle's disease have been published in the past four decades, **few have dealt with attempts at treatment, and none have documented clinically relevant improvement in exercise tolerance.**

A characteristic of McArdle's disease is a spontaneous "second-wind" phenomenon, in which the very activity that initially causes severe fatigue becomes easily tolerated after it has been continued for about 10 minutes.[11–14] The second wind is associated with a large decrease in heart rate and the level of perceived exertion.[11–13] This decrease is attributable to a substantial increase in peak oxidative capacity. The improved oxidative capacity is due to the improved delivery of extramuscular energy, particularly glucose, to working muscles, which partially compensates for the impaired glycogen breakdown.[14] **It has been known** for several decades that the **intravenous infusion of glucose** bypasses the metabolic block and can improve exercise capacity in patients with McArdle's disease.[3,14–18] The effect on exercise tolerance of **oral glucose**, which patients themselves can administer before exercise, **has not been investigated**. The effects of intravenous and oral glucose are not necessarily similar, because the absorption of glucose and the neurohormonal responses to it depend on the route of administration.[19]

Q2 In this study, we investigated whether patients with

McArdle's disease who <u>take</u> sucrose orally before exercise <u>can improve</u> work performance in the early stages of exercise—before the second wind occurs—when patients are particularly prone to muscle cramps and
50 injury. Sucrose, a disaccharide, is the most prevalent dietary sugar and is rapidly split into fructose and glucose after ingestion. Glucose and fructose bypass the metabolic block in McArdle's disease and act as equal contributors to glycolysis. We studied 12 patients with
55 McArdle's disease in a <u>single-blind</u>, <u>randomized</u>, <u>placebo-controlled</u>, <u>crossover study</u>. We tested exercise tolerance during aerobic exercise on a bicycle ergometer.

Vissing, John and Haller, Ronald G. 2003. The effect of oral sucrose on exercise tolerance in patients with McArdle's disease. *N Eng J Med* **349** (26): 2503–2509. Copyright ©2003 Massachusetts Medical Society. All rights reserved. Used with permission. RY–2006–1748.

動詞が take, improve のように現在形で使われている場合は，研究課題であることを示唆しています。この課題が今回の特定の被験者だけでなく，一般化できる重要な課題だからです。

sucrose: ショ糖
prone to: 傾向がある（see p. 14 line 59）
disaccharide: 二糖類
fructose: 果糖
ingestion: 摂取

single-blind, randomized, placebo-controlled crossover study: 単盲検無作為化プラセボ対照クロスオーバー試験（see pp. 80–81）

注意：この抜粋部分で肩付き数字で示されているのは，この論文の参考文献として原著に載せられているものです。

Lecture

Clues and patterns
A specific gap, or unknown, in medical knowledge is a clue to the authors' research aims

　どの医学論文にも，Introduction にはその論文に関する未知の医学知識の記述が書かれているはずです。それを手掛かりにすれば，著者が解き明かそうとしている問題を見つけることができます。論文の読解力は未知の部分の記述を見つけることで格段に向上します。

　In Table 8–2 (p. 75), look for patterns often used in stating a gap in the medical knowledge.

Exercise

1. Separating the known from the unknown

On each line below, write **Yes**, **No** or **unknown** to identify what was known BEFORE this research was done and what was unknown before this research was done.

_____   1. Can McArdle's disease be inherited?

_____   2. Does McArdle's disease completely block the use of glycogen in the body?

_____   3. If glucose is administered by intravenous drip, can it improve the exercise capacity in patients with McArdle's disease?

_____   4. If sucrose is taken orally, can it improve work performance in the early stages of exercise?

_____   5. Do patients with McArdle's disease often get muscle cramps and injuries if they are jogging?

_____   6. Are successful treatments available for patients with McArdle's disease?

_____   7. Are the effects of intravenous glucose and oral glucose the same?

_____   8. Do the patients of McArdle's disease usually get their muscle cramps and injuries during the early stages of exercise?

_____   9. If muscle injury occurs, does it usually happen after the second wind?

_____   10. Have many articles been written about treatment for McArdle's disease?

Lecture

What kinds of information are usually in the Introduction?

注：information という単語は複数形で使うことはありません。

　ほぼすべての論文について言えることですが，Introduction には少なくても 4 つ，時には 6 つから 8 つの種類の役立つ情報が含まれています（Table 8–1 参照）。Introduction が 1 ページ以上の長いものの場合，論文を読み慣れている人は，新しい段落への変化に注目します。段落が改められているということは，そこから研究のさらなる段階，つまり未知の部分から既知へと論理的に進んでいくことが示されているのです。

Exercises

2. Locating the various information categories in the Introduction

　In Table 8–1, write the paragraph number (1 to 4) where each kind of information is found in the Introduction to the paper on McArdle's disease. Three answers are filled in.

Table 8–1. Checklist of the main kinds of information generally found in the Introduction to a medical research paper.*

Kinds of Information	Locate the Information in our Introduction
1. The topic of the paper　この論文が扱っているテーマ	paragraph ____
Information based on other research so far: 他の研究によって今までにわかっている情報	paragraphs 1, 2 and 3
2. **Background** to the topic　この研究を始めるまでの経緯	paragraphs 1 and 2
3. **Close background** that has a direct link to this study group, or to the aims of the paper we are reading この研究グループあるいはこの論文の目的と密接に関わる背景	paragraph 3
4. **A research gap** or a statement that certain information is lacking この研究に関して未解決の情報に関する記述	paragraphs ____ and ____

(continued to the next page)

5. **The** author's **rationale**, defending the need for this study 論理的根拠（この研究の正当性）	paragraph _____
6. **The research objective**・the question or hypothesis この研究の目的（疑問または仮説）	paragraph _____
7. Potential **application or merit** of the results of this study この研究結果が応用できる可能性	paragraph _____
8. **The study type** (usually in the Methods section, but rarely in the Introduction)　研究のタイプ（通常は Methods セクションに記載されているが，まれに Introduction に書かれているときもある）	paragraph _____

* Usually 4 to 6 types of information appear in the Introduction to any medical research paper, mostly types No. 1 to No. 6 shown in this table.

3. Identify the main categories of information in the Introduction

On the line under each statement below, write the main category of information expressed in the statement (choose from this box). No. 6 has two answers.

application or merit of our results	x 1	background to the topic	x 1
the rationale	x 1	background with a close link to this study	x 2
the research objective	x 1	a gap in the research so far	x 2
the overall topic	x 1		

1. McArdle's disease is the most common disorder of muscle carbohydrate metabolism, with an estimated prevalence of about 1 case in 100,000 people.

   _____

2. Typically, the mutations ... completely block the breakdown of glycogen in muscle.

   _____

73

3. Though more than 200 articles on McArdle's disease have been published in the past four decades, few have dealt with attempts at treatment.

   _____

4. A characteristic of McArdle's disease is a spontaneous "second-wind" phenomenon. The second wind is associated with a large decrease in heart rate.

   _____

5. The effect of oral glucose on exercise tolerance has not been investigated.

   _____

6. The absorption of glucose and the neurohormonal responses to it depend on the route of administration.

   _____

   _____

7. We investigated whether patients with McArdle's disease who take sucrose orally before exercise can improve work performance in the early stages of exercise.

   _____

8. Patients themselves can administer oral glucose before exercise.

   _____

Table 8–2. Expressions commonly used in stating a gap in the research.*

Gap Statements	
· a lack of studies	· little is available on
· a paucity of material is available on	· little is known about
· **few studies have dealt with attempts at treatment**	· little has been done to clarify
· has not been clarified	· **none have documented**
· has not been determined	· not much is available on
· **has not been investigated**	· remains controversial
· has not been well documented	· remains to be solved
· is debatable	· remains unclear/ remains unknown
· is still poorly understood	· scant information is available on

* 医学雑誌では"We don't know much about McArdle's disease yet"のような日常会話的表現を見かけることはまれで，上記のような表現が使われます。

To see the Japanese translation of most of these expressions, look in this book:
Kennedy, Nell L. アクセプトされる英語医学論文を書こう！ワークショップ方式による英語の弱点克服法（菱田治子 訳）．2001, Medical View Co.: Tokyo, pp. 84–85.

4. **Recognizing the clues to a medical unknown**

From two sentences in the Introduction, write three phrases (listed in Table 8–2) that signal a gap in medical knowledge about McArdle's disease. Inside (   ), put the line number where the clue is found in this Introduction (pp. 68–70).

1. _____ have _____ with attempts at _____ .

   (lines _____ to _____)

2. _____ have _____ clinically relevant _____ in

   exercise _____ . (lines _____ to _____)

3. The effect of _____ glucose on exercise tolerance has _____

   _____ _____ . (lines _____ to _____)

75

Lecture

Is the author's argument logical and convincing?

　どの論文にも存在意義(フランス語，raison d'être)があるはずです。論文の論理的根拠は簡潔で論理的でなければなりません。そして既知の情報を基に未知の情報へと進んでいきます。マッカードル病の論文の Introduction (p. 68)では一番の論点は 35 〜 44 行目に書いてあります。

Exercise

5. Comprehension

Match the beginning of the sentence with the correct ending from the box on page 77. Write the full ending on the line.

1. Patients themselves can _____
   _____ .

2. On the other hand, the patients would have to go to the hospital _____
   _____ .

3. The effect of oral glucose _____
   _____ .

4. The authors think that oral glucose _____
   _____ .

5. Glucose administered by intravenous infusion _____
   _____ .

6. Patients with McArdle's disease are particularly prone to muscle cramps and injury_____ .

- has not been investigated
- is the same as the effect of intravenous infusion of glucose
- administer oral glucose before exercise
- in the early stages of exercise
- may improve work performance in the early stages of exercise
- bypasses the metabolic block in patients with McArdle's disease
- after they have received glucose by mouth
- give themselves the glucose by intravenous infusion
- to get an intravenous infusion

For Further Study

See the sucrose drink

The website below shows a color photograph of the sucrose drink and bicycle used in the medical research paper we are reading in Chapters 8–10. After opening the website, click "Sugar Boost Helps in McArdle's Disease."

< http://www.mda.org/publications/Quest/q112resup.html #sugar >

COLUMN

Finding the Unknown

Every medical research paper is born out of a certain <u>gap in medical knowledge</u>. In some cases, that unknown factor could make the difference between life and death.

どの医学論文も，未知の医学知識を解明する必要性から生み出されます。時には，その未知の知識が生死を分けることもあります。

Part 3: Reading the Medical Research Paper

Chapter 9 Methods・Results

The Effect of Oral Sucrose on Exercise Tolerance in Patients with McArdle's Disease

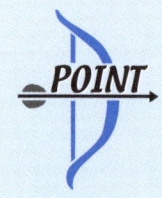

POINT
- Methods には，その研究を「いつ」「どこで」「誰が」「何を」「どのように」そして「なぜ」行ったのかが書かれています。
- Methods でも Results でも，情報は subheads（小見出し）でくくられています。Subheads を活用すれば，一語一語読まなくても必要な情報を早く見つけることができます。

Reading

CD track 23

Methods

Study population

We performed the study from April 1999 to February 2002 in 12 unrelated patients (7 men and 5 women) with McArdle's disease. Their average age was 37 years (range, 22 to 57). All the patients had a history of lifelong exercise intolerance and had had repeated episodes of cramps and myoglobinuria that were triggered by sudden vigorous exercise. Plasma lactate levels dropped slightly in response to forearm exercise. The diagnosis of McArdle's disease was confirmed in each case by a muscle biopsy that showed a lack of myophosphorylase on staining and no risidual myophosphorylase activity in skeletal muscle on biochemical testing. One patient was taking glimepiride for type 2 diabetes mellitus, but otherwise, none of the patients were taking any medications.

Study population
 = Patients or healthy volunteers who agree to participate in the medical research

were triggered by: (*Cf.* p. 3 line 42 and p. 12 line 6) [*Cf.* = compare]

biopsy: 生検

staining: 染色

residual: 残りの

myophosphorylase: 筋ホスホリラーゼ

The study was approved by the scientific ethics committee in Copenhagen, Denmark, and the institutional review board of the University of Texas Southwestern Medical Center and Presbyterian Hospital, Dallas, and all patients gave written consent.

Study design

All patients reported to the laboratory between 9 a.m. and 10 a.m. after fasting overnight. Each patient was studied on three separate days. The first day was used to define the work protocols, including a constant workload for 15 minutes on a bicycle ergometer (MedGraphics CPE 2000). On the other two days, the patients received, in random order, a caffeine-free soft drink (660 ml) that was either artificially sweetened or that contained 75 g of sucrose. The patients consumed their drinks 30 to 40 minutes before they began exercising and were unaware of the content. Interviews conducted after ingestion showed that the patients could not distinguish between the drinks. An antecubital venous catheter was inserted in each patient, and blood was periodically obtained for analysis. The heart rate was monitored continuously with a three-lead electrocardiograph.

The level of perceived exertion was scored every minute by each patient on a Borg scale,[21] in which a rating of 6 represents the least effort, and 20 the most. To investigate a possible dose-response effect, the patient with the lowest body weight was studied for an additional day, during which she consumed a drink that contained 37.5 g of sucrose (half the normal amount) before exercise.

protocol: プロトコール
ergometer: エルゴメータ

または were blinded from knowing the content (line 34)

antecubital: 肘前の (＜ ante [before] + cubital [elbow])

perceived exertion: 自覚的運動強度

dose-response effect: 用量–作用効果, 用量依存性

Statistical analysis

Blood samples were spun in a refrigerated centrifuge and stored at −20°C until analysis. Plasma glucose, lactate, pyruvate, ammonia, and free fatty acids were measured with fluorometric assays, and insulin was measured with the use of radioimmunoassay.[3] Values are reported as means ± SE. A P-value of 0.05 or lower (by two-tailed testing) was considered to indicate statistical significance. Differences in the performance of the patients after ingesting sucrose and after ingesting placebo were assessed with the use of a paired Student's *t*-test* and analysis of variance for repeated measures.

Vissing, John and Haller, Ronald G. 2003. The effect of oral sucrose on exercise tolerance in patients with McArdle's disease. *N Eng J Med* **349** (26): 2503–2509. Copyright ©2003 Massachusetts Medical Society. All rights reserved. Used with permission. RY–2006–1748.

血液の保管と解析の詳細 (line 50) は通常, 血液サンプリングの詳細 (lines 37–38) とともに書かれている。

spun: spin (回す) の過去分詞

centrifuge: 遠心分離器

pyruvate (ピルビン酸塩, 解糖代謝物の1つ) と lactate (乳酸塩) は炭水化物代謝の指標として用いられている。

are reported (現在形)

±SE: 標準誤差 (より大きな母集団から抽出された標本統計量の標準偏差, standard error)

P-value: P 値 probability

*paired *t*-test (対応のある *t* 検定) は, 同一被験者について, 時あるいは条件を変えて2回測定した場合に使用される。

Lecture

Types of study designs

Introduction の最後 (p. 70, lines 55–56) に, この研究は single-blind, randomized, placebo-controlled, crossover study (単盲検無作為化プラセボ対照クロスオーバー試験) だと書かれていました。このような情報は Introduction の最後に書かれることもまれにはありますが, 通常は Methods に書かれます。

● single-blind (単盲検): double-blind (二重盲検) では, それぞれの患者にどの治療が行われているか医師も患者も知りません。では, 単盲検の場合は医師と患者のどちらが知らされていないと思いますか。一方を選んだ理由も含めて,

英語で話し合いなさい。

- randomized（無作為化）：事前の計画はなく，無作為に選ばれる。治療の順もきまりはありません。
- placebo-controlled（プラセボ対照）：実験しようとしている治療を受けている群とプラセボ（偽薬）を受けている群を対照した研究です。通常は２つのグループで行われますが，今回の研究ではなぜ２つのグループが必要ではなかったのか，話し合いなさい。
- crossover（クロスオーバー）：２つ以上の治療を比較する方法です。最初はどちらでも任意の治療を受け，その治療が完了した後，もう片方の治療を受けます。薬物投与の場合は，初めの薬の影響が残らないよう適切な期間をおくことが必要です。

Exercise

1. Reasoning

1. In a **single**-blind study, who do you suppose would be masked from knowing which treatment was used—the patient, or the doctor? Write your answer on the lines below.

   In a ___ _____ _____ , the _____ would not be told which treatment was being used.

2. Why? With a friend, discuss your answer to the question above. Write either **the patient** or **the doctor** to complete the possible answer below:

   Because if _____ _____ was blinded to the treatment, then he (or she) may not have enough information to help _____ _____ in case something went wrong.

3. In the study on McArdle's disease, why were two groups not necessary? In English, compare your answer with a friend's answer. Complete the answer below.

In this study, two groups were not necessary because each _____ received both the _____ and the _____ . Then the results of the two different treatments were compared in each individual.

Lecture

What main information is in the Methods section? —Who, What, When, Where, How

■ WHO
この研究ではどのような人が対象になったか。

■ WHAT
どのような治療が行われたか。その結果としてどのような情報が収集できたかの概観。どの論文もまずは Introduction で投げかけられた疑問から始まり，次のステップがこの Methods のセクションに書かれている実験の概観です。

■ Approval by the Ethics Committee
この研究計画が倫理委員会で認められているという記述が必要です。マッカードル病に関するこの論文の場合，著者がコペンハーゲン（デンマーク）やダラス（アメリカ・テキサス州）の3つの研究所から参加しているため，1ヵ所からの認可では不十分です。

■ Informed Consent

インフォームド・コンセント。被験者がいる研究はすべて，各被験者から同意書をもらっていることを Methods セクションに明記しておきます。

■ WHEN, WHERE, and HOW

この研究がいつ，どこで（院内で，研究室で，等）行われたか。どのような治療がなされたか。データはどのように入手したか。ちょうど料理のレシピのように，詳しく書かれています。Methods のセクションの一つのきまりは「他のグループの被験者にまったく同じ methods で研究をできるくらい詳細な方法を記述すること」だからです。

■ Analysis

データはどのように分析されたか。データ分析の前に P-value（P 値）を決めることは，研究の一つのルールです。P 値が 0.05 なら，それが偶然に起こる可能性は 5％，つまりグループ間に違いがなければ，起こる可能性は 20 件に 1 つということになります。P 値が 0.001 ならその確率は 1000 分の 1 です。

Exercises

2. Using the Subheads

This Methods information (pp. 78–80) is divided into three categories:

　　Study population　　　Study design　　　Statistical analysis

Write one subhead that would help us find each type of information below.

1. exactly how the sucrose was used　　　＿＿＿＿＿＿＿＿＿＿＿＿

2. the age of the oldest patient　　　＿＿＿＿＿＿＿＿＿＿＿＿

3. the number of women participants _____

4. whether blood tests were made _____

5. what time the patients started _____

6. whether any patients had other illnesses _____

7. exercise duration _____

8. how the heart rate was measured _____

9. whether breakfast was allowed before exercise _____

10. how comparisons were measured _____

3. **Comprehension**

   Choose one answer for each question; write A, B, or C on the line.

   1. **The purpose of the interview was _____ .**
      A. to find out whether any of the patients were allergic to the drink
      B. to show the patients how to do the experiments
      C. to find out whether the patients could detect the difference between the drinks

   2. **During exercise, _____ .**
      A. a forearm catheter was inserted into each patient's arm
      B. a blood sample was taken from the patient and the heart rate was measured
      C. a tissue sample was taken by muscle biopsy and stored at −20°C until biochemical analysis and staining

3. In patients with McArdle's disease, this study _____ .

   A. compared the effects of oral sucrose with the effects of intravenous infusion of sucrose

   B. compared the effects of a drink containing sucrose with the effects of a drink containing artificial sweetener

   C. compared the effects of sucrose ingestion in men patients with the effects of sucrose ingestion in women patients

4. The placebo was _____ .

   A. a drink containing 75 grams of sucrose

   B. a drink containing 37.5 grams of sucrose

   C. a drink containing an artificial sweetener

4. Say the Professional Expresssion

臨床研究について書く場合，著者も編者も言葉を慎重に使っています。注意していれば，批判を受けることも，また医療過誤の非難を受けることも避けられるからです。

一人が **Table 9–1** の右側を隠して，左側の表現を順不同に **1** つずつ読み，もう一人がそれに対応する専門的表現を答えなさい。[ペアワーク]

Table 9–1. Professional expressions compared with nonprofessional expressions.

Nonprofessional Expressions	Professional Expressions
12 **patients were used**	12 patients participated in the study 12 patients took part in the trial 12 patients were tested for ...
Experiments were conducted **on** 12 **patients**	We performed the study in 12 patients The study was performed in 12 patients
The patients **were made to** drink a ...	The patients received a soft drink ... The patients were given a soft drink ...
We **made the patients sign** their consent	All patients gave written consent All patients provided written consent Written consent was received from all patients

Reading

Results

Heart rate, level of perceived exertion, and workload

After ingestion of the placebo drink, the mean peak heart rate (156 ± 3 beats per minute) and level of perceived exertion (15.9 ± 0.5) occurred in the seventh minute of exercise (Fig. 1) and were followed by a spontaneous second wind, with a drop in the heart rate of 35 ± 3 beats per minute ($P<0.001$). After patients ingested sucrose, however, the heart rate in the seventh minute of exercise was 34 ± 3 beats per minute lower than at the same time during exercise after ingestion of placebo ($P<0.001$) (Fig. 1) and the patients did not have a second wind. Accordingly, perceived exertion in the seventh minute of exercise was considerably lower after the ingestion of sucrose than after the ingestion of placebo ($P<0.001$). In four patients who received placebo supplementation and who had received sucrose in their first trial, the workload had to be decreased slightly for approximately five minutes before the second wind occurred (Fig. 1), because of the patients' near-exhaustion and the risk of muscle injury.

In the one patient in whom half the normal dose of sucrose was tested, the peak heart rate in the seventh minute of exercise was 164 beats per minute after she ingested placebo, 142 after the ingestion of 37.5 g of sucrose, and 116 after the ingestion of 75 g of sucrose. The second-wind phenomenon was obliterated by the high dose of sucrose but (was) only blunted by the lower dose (Fig. 2).

CD track 24

2ヵ所の下線部について反対の条件下での結果を見つけなさい。

perceived exertion: 自覚的運動

15.9 ± 0.5: ［読み方］ fifteen point nine plus-or-minus zero point five

ingested: 摂取した

was obliterated: 消される

(was) blunted: 鈍らされる

Plasma levels of glucose, insulin, lactate, pyruvate, ammonia, and free fatty acids

<u>Sucrose ingestion</u> resulted in marked hyperinsulinemia and an increase in the plasma glucose level that was 36 mg per deciliter (2.0 mmol per liter) greater than the level <u>after patients ingested placebo</u>. Both increases were maintained throughout the exercise period (P<0.005). In line with the increased availability of glucose, plasma levels of lactate and pyruvate were elevated at rest after the ingestion of sucrose. Plasma glucose, lactate, and insulin levels all fell during exercise under both conditions. The exercise-induced increase in plasma ammonia* was attenuated, and the availability of free fatty acids, as inferred from the plasma levels of free fatty acids, decreased with sucrose.

Vissing, John and Haller, Ronald G. 2003. The effect of oral sucrose on exercise tolerance in patients with McArdle's disease. *N Eng J Med* **349** (26): 2503–2509. Copyright ©2003 Massachusetts Medical Society. All rights reserved. Used with permission. RY-2006-1748.

marked: 著明な，顕著な

hyperinsulinemia: 高インスリン血症

in line with: 一致して

both conditions (see lines 30 and 33)

induce (see p. 95, line 38)

was attenuated: 弱められた

* 運動中のエネルギー状態の直接的指標として，血漿中のアンモニア濃度が用いられている。

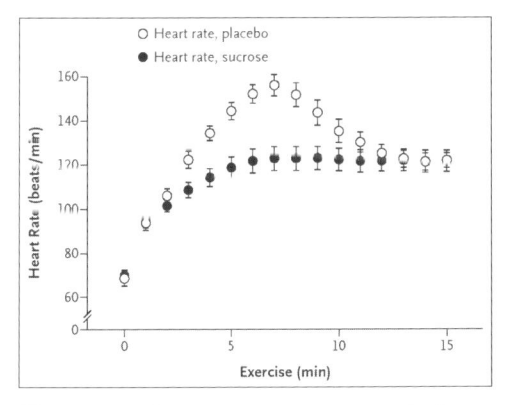

Figure 1. Heart-rate response during cycle exercise in the patients with McArdle's disease. Each person ingested either a placebo drink or a drink with 75 g of sucrose 30 to 40 minutes before exercise.

Copyright ©2003 Massachusetts Medical Society. All rights reserved. Adapted with permission Nov. 2005. RY-2006-1748.

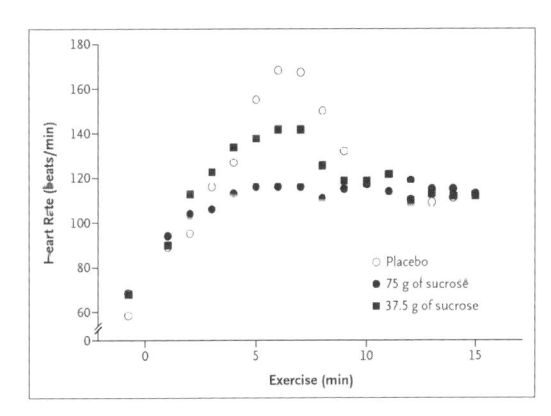

Figure 2. Heart-rate response during cycle exercise in the patient with the lowest body weight. This woman was 31 years of age.

Used with permission, RY-2006-1748.

Lecture

What main information is in the Results section?

■ The bare data

　Resultsセクションは論文の流れの第3段階です。Introductionで投げかけた疑問に対してMethodsで述べられた実験が行われ、Resultsではその結果が解釈を加えず生のデータで示されます。

■ Visual comparison

　表やグラフは、そのデータの関係がすぐにわかるよう、また容易に比較ができるようにするためのものです。

■ Statistics

　P値はデータ結果が偶然で起こったものでないことを明示します。

Exercises

5. Comparing the Methods and Results

　To complete each sentence below, write one word on each line. Then, in the box write <u>Methods</u> or <u>Results</u> to tell which section contains the answer.

[Caution: Method<u>s</u>, not Method; and Result<u>s</u>, not Result]

1. The youngest patient in this study was _____ years old.

2. The study included _____ men and _____ women.

3. In patients _____ sucrose, the heart rate in the seventh minute of exercise was 34 ± 3 beats per minute _____ than at the same time during exercise after _____ of placebo.

4. One of the patients was _____ medication for type 2 _____ mellitus.

5. In an extra part of this study, one patient consumed half the _____ amount of sucrose.

6. In the patient receiving half the _____ dose of sucrose, the peak heart rate in the seventh minute of exercise was _____ beats per minute after she ingested placebo, _____ after the _____ of 37.5 grams of sucrose, and _____ after the _____ of 75 grams of sucrose.

6. **True or False**

On each line write **True** or **False**, and in the box write either **Methods** or **Results**, according to which section the answer is in.

_____ 1. In one patient with low body weight, the low dose of sucrose did not stop the second-wind phenomenon.

_____ 2. After the patients ingested placebo, the peak heart rate occurred in the seventh minute of exercise.

_____ 3. Each patient was tested for about three years, from April 1999 to February 2002.

_____ 4. The patients were not told the protocol.

_____ 5. One patient was given half the normal dose of sucrose to test whether the effect would depend on the dose.

_____ 6. Each patient participated in the study for a minimum of three days.

_____ 7. In four patients, the workload was reduced during the cycling exercise because they were getting tired.

_____ 8. The workload was reduced in four patients during the cycling exercise because they injured their muscles.

7. **Reviewing the Introduction, Methods, Results**

Choose the single best answer to each question below, according to this paper. Write A, B, C or D.

1. In this study, _____ .

    A. seven patients took the placebo only, and five took the sucrose drink
    B. five patients took the placebo only, and seven took the sucrose drink
    C. both drinks were consumed by each patient, though not in the same order
    D. all the patients consumed the sucrose drink first, then the placebo

2. If the doctors in a study knew which drink each patient was given but the patients did not know, this kind of study would be _____ .

   A. a double-blind study

   B. a single-blind study

   C. a crossover study

   D. a randomized study

3. If neither the doctors nor the patients were told which drink was given, the type of study would be _____ .

   A. a double-blind study

   B. a single-blind study

   C. a crossover study

   D. a randomized study

4. In the Methods section, the verbs are mostly in _____ . This signals a specific procedure at a specific hospital or testing center, and not a general principle.

   A. the present tense（現在形）

   B. the past tense（過去形）

   C. the present progressive tense（現在進行形 ...ing）

   D. none of the above

5. In the Results section, the verbs are mostly in _____ . This signals the readers that that sentence is about a result of the study described in the paper they are reading now, and is not necessarily a general principle for other patients yet.

   A. the present tense（現在形）

   B. the past tense（過去形）

   C. the present progressive tense（現在進行形 ...ing）

   D. none of the above

8. Comparing figures and text

Choose the one correct answer to each question below. Write A, B, C or D.

1. The text of _____ mentions certain figures by the figure number.

    A. the Abstract
    B. the Introduction
    C. the Methods
    D. the Results

2. In Figure 1, each open circle (○) represents _____ .

    A. one patient after that patient consumed the placebo drink
    B. one patient after that patient consumed the sucrose drink
    C. all 12 patients after they consumed the placebo drink
    D. all 12 patients after they consumed the sucrose drink

3. In Figure 1, each closed circle (●) represents _____ .

    A. one patient after that patient consumed the placebo drink
    B. one patient after that patient consumed the sucrose drink
    C. all 12 patients after they consumed the placebo drink
    D. all 12 patients after they consumed the sucrose drink

4. Seven minutes after starting the exercise, patients who ingested the sucrose drink had an average heart rate of _____ .

    A. about 34 beats per minute
    B. about 122 beats per minute
    C. about 142 beats per minute
    D. about 156 beats per minute

5. Figure 2 shows that, in the seventh minute of exercise, this patient's lowest heart rate was achieved _____ .

    A. after consuming the placebo

    B. after consuming 75 grams of sucrose

    C. after consuming 34 grams of sucrose

    D. none of the answers above

6. Figure 2 shows that, in the seventh minute of exercise, _____ .

    A. the effect of the placebo may depend on the amount ingested

    B. the effect of the placebo depends on the amount ingested

    C. the effect of sucrose may depend on the amount ingested

    D. for sure, the effect of sucrose depends on the amount ingested

For Further Study

A quick guide

Table 9–2. Symbols and abbreviations commonly seen in the Results.*

Symbol or Abbreviation	Reading	Symbol or Abbreviation	Reading
>	greater than	CBC	complete blood (cell) count
<	less than	RBC	red blood (cell) count
≥	greater than or equal to	WBC	white blood (cell) count
≤	less than or equal to	ECG, EKG	electrocardiogram
≠	not equal to	α, β	alpha, beta
10-fold	ten times（10 倍）	γ, μ	gamma, micro
mm Hg	millimeters of mercury	♂, ♀	male, female
e.g.	for example	30 ± 2 h	thirty plus/minus two hours
i.e.	that is, namely	~ 7 in.	approximately seven inches
viz.	namely	1.34 lb = 500 g	1 point 34 pounds = 500 grams
37 °C = 98.6 °F	37 degrees Centigrade (Celsius) equals 98 point 6 degrees Fahrenheit	1 oz = ~ 30 g (31.103 g)	1 ounce is approximately equal to 30 grams
vs, vs.	versus	ENT	ear, nose, throat（耳鼻咽喉科）

*In addition, see Table 11–1 (p. 117)

Part 3: Reading the Medical Research Paper

Chapter 10 Discussion

The Effect of Oral Sucrose on Exercise Tolerance in Patients with McArdle's Disease

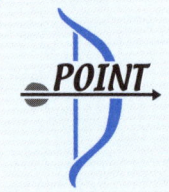

POINT
- Discussion は，著者が研究を終了した後，その正当性を述べるところです。
- 研究結果が，最初に立てた仮説の裏づけになっていますか。

Reading

CD track 25

Discussion

1　In this study, sucrose ingestion before exercise markedly improved exercise tolerance in all the patients with McArdle's disease.

Patients with McArdle's disease have an inability to
5　break down muscle glycogen. The oxidative limitation is most severe in the first seven to eight minutes of exercise. During this period, moderate exercise, such as brisk walking, may provoke muscle cramping and injury in these patients.[14]

10　No treatment has yet been found that can alleviate symptoms, improve exercise tolerance, and provide protection against muscle injury during the early minutes of exercise in patients with McArdle's disease.[22–24] Treatment with high-protein diet or creatine supple-
15　mentation has never been translated into clinically meaningful responses in these patients.[22–24] Attempts to boost energy metabolism within the muscles and

---

Most Discussions open with a statement of the main finding.

provoke: 引き起こす

alleviate: 緩和する
symptoms: 症状

creatine supplementation: クレアチン補充

translated: 翻訳された

thus boost exercise tolerance in such patients by treatment with creatine or branched-chain amino acids have also failed.[25–28] Transfer of the intact myophosphorylase gene to myophosphorylase-deficient muscle has been performed in vitro with some success,[29,30] but this approach requires much more investigation before it can be considered for clinical use. Meanwhile, treatments need to be developed that can minimize the incidence of muscle injury and increase exercise tolerance in patients with McArdle's disease.

Our study **provides** evidence that sucrose ingestion before exercise markedly **improves** exercise tolerance in patients with McArdle's disease. The treatment is effective only during the time when patients are highly susceptible to muscle injury—that is, during the first minutes of exercise, when there is a low availability of bloodborne fuels plus an absence of glycogen-derived pyruvate. Treatment with sucrose virtually abolishes the spontaneous second-wind phenomenon, because the increased availability of glucose at the onset of exercise effectively induces a second wind from the start of exercise. The treatment seems to cause a markedly lower level of perceived exertion on the Borg scale and a dramatic lowering of the heart rate that is directly attributable to an increase in the oxidative capacity of the muscles.[14]

The clinical relevance of the treatment is emphasized by the fact that the participants have continued to use the treatment one to seven times a week, with consistent improvement in exercise tolerance. The treatment with sucrose should help prevent muscle injury by augmenting the oxidative capacity of the muscles, thus increasing the threshold of exercise necessary to induce muscle injury.

Although the simple treatment we propose may be the single most effective treatment for patients with McArdle's disease, **it has limitations**. The treatment is not suited for situations that require unexpected vigorous exercise. Furthermore, the effect of the treatment is short-lived and therefore unlikely to affect endurance during long-term exercise. Repeated doses of oral glucose may lead to an intake of calories that exceeds expenditure, and would inhibit the use of free fatty acids, which is an important fuel source during prolonged exercise. The treatment is unlikely to be helpful in static exercise such as weight lifting, during which blood flow to working muscles is curtailed. Treatment with sucrose would usually be contraindicated in persons with diabetes mellitus, although we found it to be as effective in one patient with type 2 diabetes mellitus as it was in other patients.

One patient not included in the study reported using oral sucrose loading and had developed a "soft-drink addiction" that had resulted in substantial weight gain. This anecdotal experience emphasizes the importance of informing patients with McArdle's disease that they should ingest sucrose only before engaging in exercise that is known from experience to elicit muscle symptoms.

We administered sucrose 30 to 40 minutes before exercise to ensure that sufficient amounts of glucose and fructose were absorbed from the intestine. However, subsequent reports from our patients indicate that an interval of 15 minutes between consumption and exercise may suffice. Whether the amount of ingested sucrose should be adjusted to body weight is not clear. However, the attenuated effect of half a dose of sucrose on exercise tolerance in the patient with the lowest body weight suggests that **this question warrants investigation**.

This study **shows** that, in patients with McArdle's disease, oral sucrose ingested before exercise alleviates the muscle symptoms and abolishes the second-wind phenomenon that occurs during the early stages of exercise, when patients are prone to muscle injury. When informing patients with McArdle's disease about such treatment, doctors should stress the importance of restricting its use to avoid unintentional weight gain.

* Vissing, John and Haller, Ronald G. 2003. The effect of oral sucrose on exercise tolerance in patients with McArdle's disease. *N Eng J Med* **349** (26): 2503–2509. Copyright ©2003 Massachusetts Medical Society. All rights reserved. Used with permission. RY–2006–1748.

warrant: 是認する

← The authors' answer to the research problem stated in the Introduction (p. 69, lines 45–50)

prone to: 傾向がある (See p. 14, line 59)

* For the physiological defense, see the full Discussion in the original Journal.

注意：この抜粋部分で肩付き数字で示されているのは，この論文の参考文献として原著に載せられているものです。

Lecture

Clues to Reading the Discussion

■ 過去形の動詞

Discussion で<u>過去形</u>の動詞が使われていれば，それが（a）その論文の<u>結果</u>か，（b）以前に他の人が行った研究<u>結果</u>かのいずれかについての記述だとわかります。

Past tense

■ 現在形の動詞

<u>現在形</u>の動詞が使われている記述は，世界中のどの医師や患者にも当てはめることができる<u>一般的</u>なものであったり，<u>解釈</u>であることがわかります。

Present tense

Exercises

1. **Interpretation of the results**

   Choose the single best generalization as the answer to each question below, according to this paper. Write A, B, C, or D on the line.

   1. If the patients do not exercise after ingesting sucrose, _____ .
      A. their exercise tolerance will have greater improvement
      B. they have a higher risk of muscle injury
      C. they may gain weight
      D. their pain will become more severe

   2. For patients with McArdle's disease, _____ .
      A. this paper offers little hope
      B. taking sucrose orally is an attractive possibility
      C. gene therapy is currently the best treatment
      D. receiving sucrose intravenously can give the greatest help

   3. In McArdle's disease, _____ .
      A. it is difficult for researchers to find enough patients
      B. because the muscles cannot store glycogen, they cannot use glucose as fuel for exercise
      C. sucrose ingestion can cure the disease in about 25 percent of the patients
      D. though the muscles cannot store glycogen, they can use glucose as fuel for exercise

   4. For McArdle's disease, _____ .
      A. gene therapy is the only cure
      B. gene therapy is the only cure, but it has not been approved by the government because people are afraid to use it
      C. gene therapy takes a long time to take effect, but sucrose takes effect in a few minutes
      D. gene therapy is expected to be the treatment of choice in the future

5. In McArdle's disease, _____ .

   A. sucrose ingestion prevents muscle injury and increases the heart rate during exercise

   B. sucrose ingestion improves the patient's tolerance for exercise and reduces the risk of muscle injury

   C. sucrose ingestion is an inexpensive cure that the patients can do for themselves without hospital intervention

   D. sucrose ingestion is recommended without exercise if the patient wishes to gain weight

6. The focus of this research was on _____ .

   A. diagnosis
   B. pain evaluation
   C. rehabilitation
   D. treatment

2. **Comprehension**

   On each line, write **True** or **False**.

   _____ 1. Oral sucrose has a good long-lasting effect.

   _____ 2. The results of this study are in agreement with the authors' hypothesis.

   _____ 3. After completing this study, some of these patients wanted to use the sucrose drink at home every week by themselves.

   _____ 4. In the beginning, the patients wore a blindfold over their eyes.

   _____ 5. The doctor was allowed to see the patients' names at any time.

   _____ 6. If sucrose is taken 30-to-40 minutes before exercise, the patients are protected from almost any kind of exercise.

Lecture

What is the function of the Discussion?

■ Discussion の役割

　Results セクションでは生のデータがそのまま示されますが，Discussion セクションでは，下記の3点が示されます。

　①要となる結果の解釈，

　②今回得られた新しい結果とそれまでの他の研究との関連，

　　i. 研究結果が一致するのか一致しないのか

　　ii. 他の研究結果と一致しない場合の考えられる理由

　③今回の新しい結果を臨床の場でどのように応用できるか。

　ここで重要なことは，著者がまだ教科書に記載されていない発見をし，医学の知識に新しい事実を加えたということです。また通常，Discussion ではさらなる研究が必要な別の視点の問題が明らかにされるという点が大変重要です。よって読者は誰でもその研究をし，論文を書く可能性があります。

　マッカードル病の治療法はまだ見つかっていないため，患者さんの多くは腎不全になり，亡くなっていきます。しかし，その問題を解決し，世界中の患者さんを助けるために医学研究者と臨床医をより近づける新しい決定的なつながりを発見する次の著者に私たちの誰かがならないともかぎりません。

■ What questions should we ask?

　Discussion セクションを読んだ後，以下の2つを自分に問いかけなさい。

　①今回の研究で明らかになったことを基にさらに積み上げていくには，どのような研究をする必要があるか。

　②今回の研究でどのような問題が提起されたか。

Exercises

3. Comprehension

以下の文のそれぞれの空所に当てはまる最適な答を A–E から選び，文を完成させなさい。

1. According to the authors, two points that ought to be studied further are _____ and _____ .

    A. the amount of time the patient should wait between consuming the drink and doing exercise
    B. whether this treatment is also effective for weight-lifting exercise
    C. whether changing the taste of the drink would affect the results
    D. whether the amount of the sucrose ought to be based on the patient's body weight
    E. whether men require larger amounts of the drink than women do

4. Using the genetics code

下に示す記号（Code）に従って，それぞれの記述に合うよう，□や○を塗りなさい。

注：□や○に斜線が書いてある場合（▨ ⦸）は死亡したことを示します。

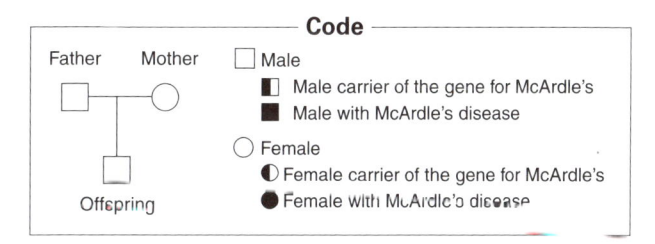

1. The father has McArdle's disease, and the mother is healthy but she is a carrier. Their daughter (their firstborn) is a carrier, and their son has McArdle's disease.

2. The father and mother are both carriers. Their son, who is their firstborn, is a carrier, and their daughter is normal and completely disease-free.

COLUMN

Autosomal Recessive Genetic Disorder

McArdle's disease is autosomal recessive. That means it is caused by an error in a single DNA gene. Autosomal means the error occurs on chromsome 1-to-22 rather than on the 23rd sex-linked X chromosome. Recessive diseases are diseases where both copies of a gene must be damaged, or mutated. Generally this means that, to have the disease, the child must inherit a bad copy of the gene from both parents. Except for rare exceptions, the patterns of inheritance tend to be as follows:

マッカードル病は常染色体劣性疾患で，1つのDNA遺伝子の変異が原因で起こります。Autosomal（常染色体性）とは，性と関連する23番目のX染色体ではなく，1～22染色体に変異が起こることを意味します。Recessive（劣性遺伝）の疾患とは，遺伝子の複製時に両方とも損傷を負っているか変異を起こしているかどちらかです。通常，劣性遺伝の疾患が起こるということは，子供が父母両方から正常でない遺伝子を受け継ぐという意味です。まれな場合を除いて，遺伝のパターンには次のような傾向がみられます。

1. A person with McArdle's disease has two bad copies of the gene. Therefore, if the affected person marries an unaffected, normal person, their child will receive one bad copy of the gene from the affected parent and one good copy from the unaffected parent. This means the child will be a carrier.

2. A carrier does not usually have the disease or the symptoms because the good gene from the other parent can make up for the bad copy and maintain health.

3. If a person with McArdle's disease marries a carrier, the odds are 100% that the child will be a carrier and a 50% chance the child will inherit the disease.

4. If a carrier marries a carrier, their child has a 25% chance of having the disease, a 50% chance of being a carrier, and a 25% chance of being neither diseased nor a carrier. The situation where both parents are carriers is the most likely way that children are born with the disease.

5. If one parent is a carrier and the other is unaffected, the child cannot get the disease, but has a 50% chance of being a carrier.

6. An autosomal disease affects male and female offspring in fairly equal numbers. This is because autosomal refers to the non-sex chromosomes 1-to-22, not the X-linked sex chromosomes.

5. Autosomal recessive genetic disorder

102 ページの Column で説明されている autosomal recessive genetic disorder（常染色体劣性遺伝性疾患）の傾向に従い，次の 20 家族のうち，どの家族が **likely**（可能性がある）で，どの家族が **unlikely**（可能性がない）か，それぞれの線上に書きなさい。

注：家族の中に一人でも可能性のない子供がいる場合，答えは unlikely になります。

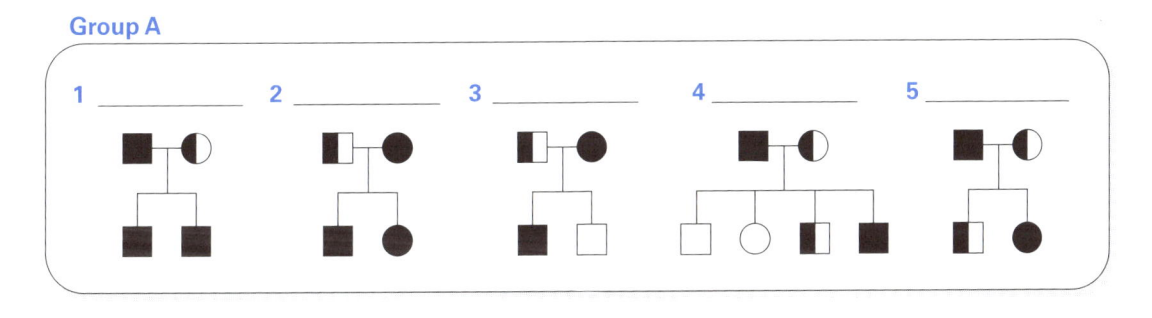

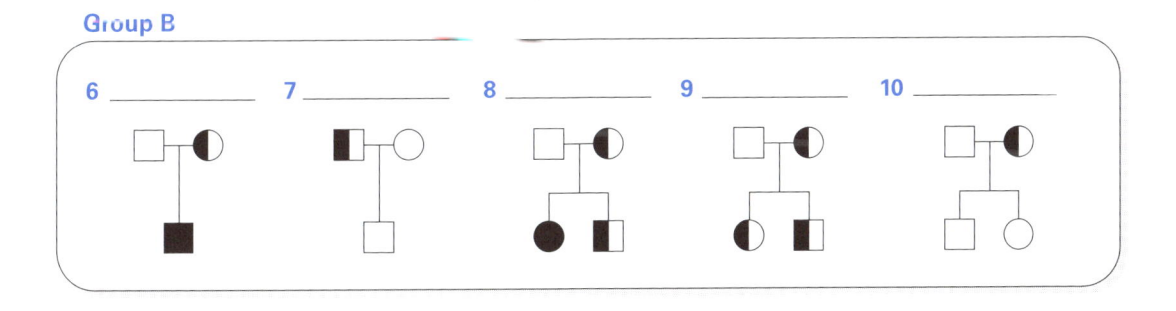

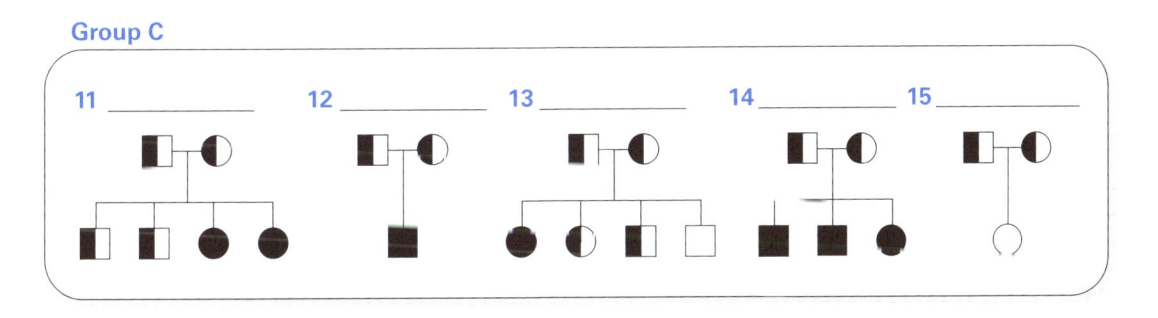

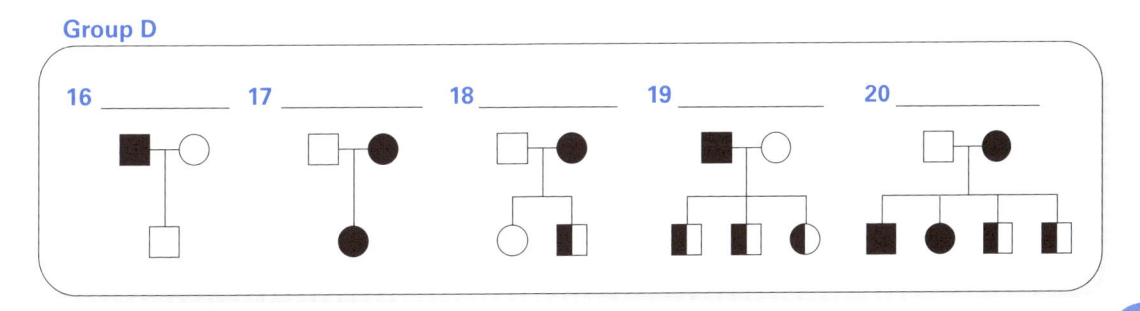

Group A

1 _____ 2 _____ 3 _____ 4 _____ 5 _____

Group B

6 _____ 7 _____ 8 _____ 9 _____ 10 _____

Group C

11 _____ 12 _____ 13 _____ 14 _____ 15 _____

Group D

16 _____ 17 _____ 18 _____ 19 _____ 20 _____

6. Overview of the Discussion

Number each paragraph of the Discussion (pp. 94–97). From the box below, match each topic with the paragraph where that topic is discussed.

1. _____   2. _____   3. _____   4. _____   5. _____

6. _____   7. _____   8. _____   9. _____

> A. Caution
> B. Defense for the clinical use of the sucrose treatment
> C. Conclusion (present tense, generalized for all patients with this disease)
> D. The authors' solution in generalizable terms, with physiological defense
> E. Comment on other treatments
> F. Limitations of this treatment
> G. The problem
> H. Main result of the present research
> I. An angle that requires further study

For Further Study

"The Effect of Oral Sucrose on Exercise Tolerance in Patients with McArdle's Disease" を読んだ後, あるボストンの医師が a Letter to the Editor に手紙を書き, ショ糖の代わりにコーンスターチを使ってはどうか, そうすれば体重の増加を招くこともなくより安全ではないか, と提案しました。

それに対し著者の Dr. Vissing と Dr. Haller は, コーンスターチは glycogen storage disease の1型 (Type I) には良いかもしれないが, 5型 (Type V) のマッカードル病には良くない, と答え, 簡潔にその理由を説明しました。この手紙のやり取りは, 原著が掲載された3ヵ月半後の *New England Journal of*

cornstarch: コーンスターチ
（トウモロコシのデンプン）

McArdle's disease is known also as glycogen storage disease type V, and as muscle glycogen phosphorylase deficiency.

Medicine の終わりに近い Correspondence のセクションに掲載されています［*N Eng J Med* 2004; 350(15): 1575–1576］。

このように読者と著者は自由なやり取りをするなかで，協力して新しい理論や証拠を積み上げていけるのです。誌上での手紙のやり取りは，医学論文の Discussion の延長のようなものです。このような略式の Discussion をも利用して，医師たちはお互いに切磋琢磨して真実を追求していきます。このようにして臨床的に根拠のある事実の探求はずっと継続されてゆくのです。

論文は，たくさん読めば読むほど簡単に読めるようになります。

Exercises

7. Review the beginning, middle and end of the medical research paper

In ANY research paper, first, read the sentence in these three shaded areas.

The authors choose a science problem from the world

1. General topic
2. Problem

Introduction — Introduction
Methods — Methods
Local laboratory
Results — Results
Discussion — Discussion

3. Answer

Gives the answer to the world

- The **Introduction** shows the problem before this paper was published.
  (The objective of this paper is …)
  (The objective of this study was …)

- The **Methods** explains what the authors did and how, to find a solution.
  (The verbs are in the past tense)

- The **Results** tells what the authors found.
  (The verbs are in the past tense)

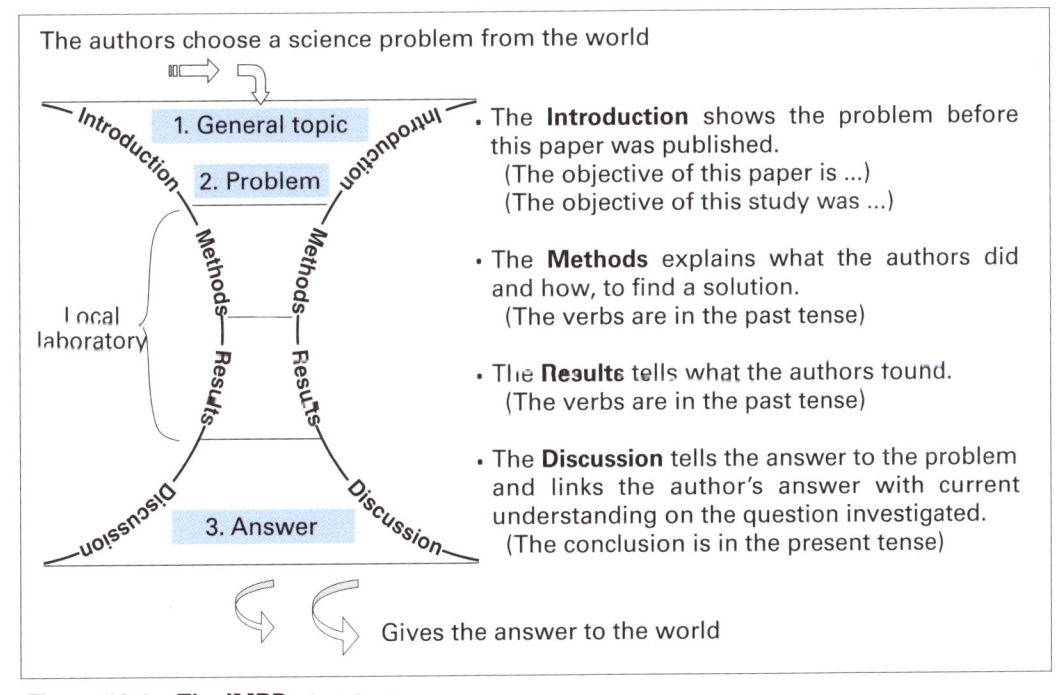

- The **Discussion** tells the answer to the problem and links the author's answer with current understanding on the question investigated.
  (The conclusion is in the present tense)

Figure 10.1. The IMRD structure.

The Introduction **receives** an idea from the broad world of science, isolates a particular problem, and narrows it down to the facet that the authors of that paper are investigating. The Discussion **gives back** to the world of science the answer these authors find to that problem.

8. Review the IMRD structure and function

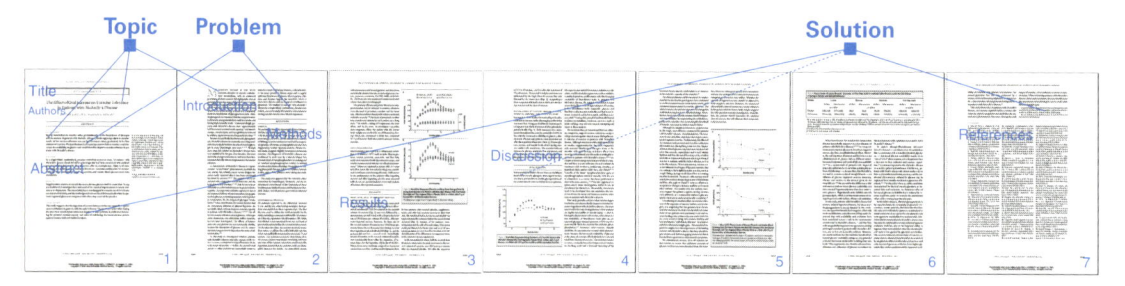

Figure 10.2

Write A, B, or C on the line.

1. The Introduction starts with a statement about _____ .

    A. the objective of this research

    B. a general phenomenon regarding the topic of this research

    C. the author's previous paper

2. The Introduction often ends with a statement about _____ .

    A. the objective of this research

    B. a general phenomenon regarding the topic of this research

    C. the author's previous paper

3. The Discussion _____ .

    A. interprets the results of the study

    B. repeats the results of the study

    C. tells how the main result was found

Write **Introduction**, **Methods**, **Results**, or **Discussion** on the line.

4. Graphs are part of the _____ section.

5. In the _____ , the authors justify their results, explaining why such results may have happened.

6. In the _____ , the authors explain the rationale behind their hypothesis.

Part 4
Reading the Case Report

Part 4: Reading the Case Report

Chapter 11. Case Report: A 33-year-old Woman with Abdominal Pain, Vomiting, and Erythema

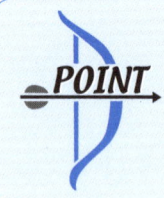

POINT
- 患者に何が起こったか。
- これらの出来事の時間経過はどうであったか。
- 医師は，なぜそのような処置を取ったのか。

Lecture

The formal case report

Chapters 8–10 でみた医学論文とは逆に，論文として発表された症例報告 (case report) では身体所見や検査結果の記載の後に疾患名がでてくることがあります。その場合は，最初に，現れている症状や病歴を考え，診断名を推測しながら進むというやり方で，読者は診断をする過程に入っていきます。

Reading

CD track 26

Case report

1 A 33-year-old woman was admitted to our hospital because of upper abdominal pain, vomiting, polyarthralgia, and erythema. The patient had been in generally
5 good health, but when she was 27, morning stiffness

polyarthralgia: 多発関節痛
erythema: 紅斑

and, on motion, pain over the right elbow developed and gradually progressed to bilateral involvement of the hand, knee, foot, and the proximal interphalangeal (PIP) and distal interphalangeal (DIP) joints. At 29, she was found to have Raynaud's phenomenon and sclerodactylia, but both disorders resolved spontaneously in 2 years. At 30, she had an appendectomy, and high fever lasted for 8 days after the operation. In January 2005, a month before admission, she had high fever; swelling of the right cervical lymph nodes; and localized edema on the forehead, eyelids, and legs. These symptoms resolved in 3 days without therapy. In February 2005, she was admitted to our hospital (present admission). She is not married, and her parents and five siblings are in excellent health.

Physical examination revealed erythema multiforme (discoid rash) on the chest, palms and back (Fig. 1); conjunctival injection; angioneurotic edema on the forehead, chin, and flexor surfaces of the forearms; and polyarthritis involving both hands, both elbows, and the right foot. Uncorrected visual acuity is 20/40 in the right eye and 20/30 in the left eye. Corrected visual acuity is 20/20 in the right eye and 20/30 in the left eye. Results of other physical examinations were normal except for slight pressure pain on the abdomen.

Results of blood chemical laboratory studies as well as the upper gastrointestinal roentgenograms were normal. In addition, the feces tested negative for occult blood, and the urine contained no protein and few casts. Hematologic and immunologic laboratory tests showed that no lupus erythematosus cells were present, but the

bilateral: 両側性の，左右の

proximal: 近位の

interphalangeal: 指節間の

distal: 遠位の

Raynaud's phenomenon: レーノー現象

sclerodactylia: 強指症，手指（足指）硬化症

resolve: 消散する

appendectomy: 虫垂切除術

cervical: 頸〔部〕の

edema: 浮腫，水腫

siblings: きょうだい（男女の区別をつけない兄弟姉妹。英語では5 siblings というと，本人以外に5人のきょうだいがいるという意味）

erythema multiforme: 多形性紅斑

conjunctival injection: 結膜充血

angioneurotic: 血管運動神経性の

flexor surfaces: 屈側面

polyarthritis: 多発性関節炎

visual acuity: 視力

20/20: ［読み方］twenty-twenty

roentgenograms: commonly called X-ray images, X-ray pictures

occult blood: 潜血

casts: 円柱（腎疾患の尿細管でつくられ，尿中に出現する柱状のもの）

serum tested positive for antinuclear antibody (ANA) at a dilution of 1:1,024. Cellular immunity indicators such as T cells, B cells and stimulation index with phytohemagglutinin were within normal range. In serum analyses for complement, serum C3 was 20 mg/dL, CH50 was 11 U/mL (normal range is 33-61 U/mL), and the serum tested positive for C1q precipitins of the low molecular weight type.

antinuclear antibody: 抗核抗体

phytohemagglutinin: フィトヘムアグルチニン (PHA)

complement: 補体

mg/dL: ［読み方］milligrams per deciliter

U/mL: ［読み方］units per milliliter

C1q precipitins: C1q 沈降素（C1qは補体の一種）

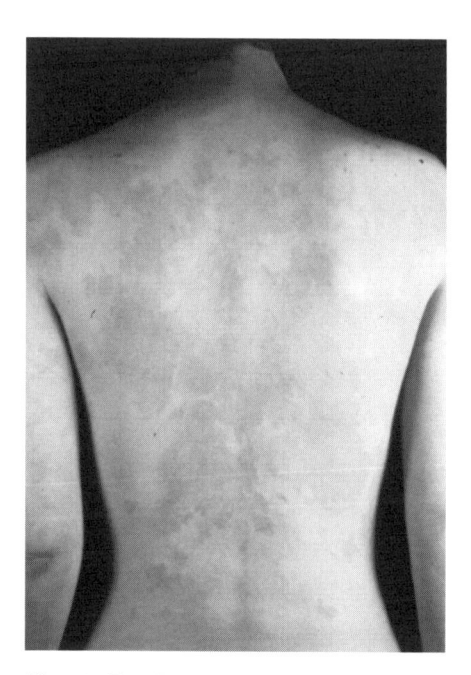

Fig. 1. Erythema multiforme on the back.

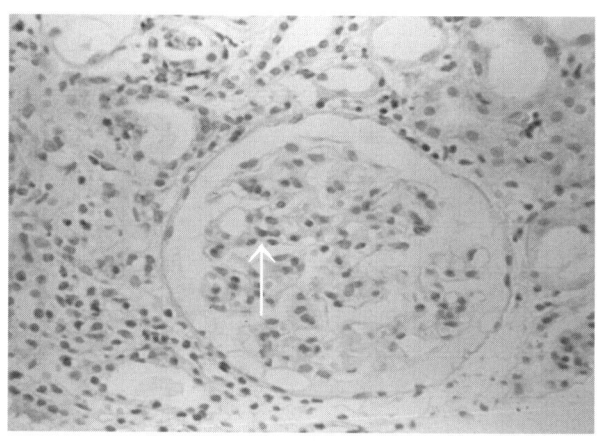

Fig. 2. Histological findings in the kidney biopsy specimen.
Slight proliferation of mesangial cells suggests a minimal renal change.

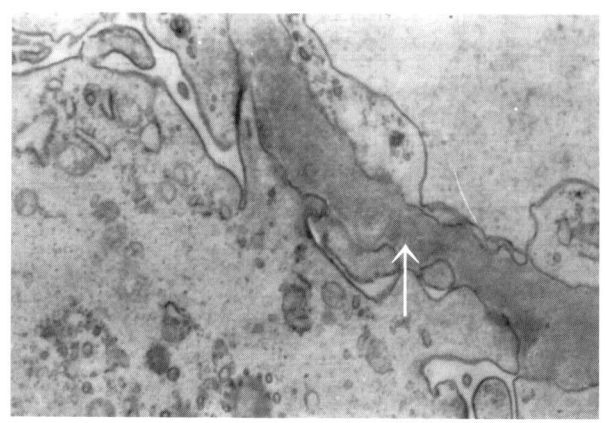

Fig. 3. Ultrastructure of the kidney biopsy specimen.
Electron microscopy disclosed homogeneous granular deposits in the subepithelium. These deposits were interpreted as an indication of slight membranous nephropathy.

In March 2005 (one month after admission), swelling appeared in the right cervical and right axillary lymph nodes, and the biopsy specimen showed chronic lymphadenitis. A renal biopsy specimen disclosed slight proliferation of mesangial cells (Fig. 2) and subepithelial deposits (Fig. 3).

Diagnosis and therapeutic intervention

Our diagnosis was a systemic lupus erythematosus (SLE)-related syndrome with special reference to hypocomplementemia and the presence of circulating C1q precipitins. This is classified as incomplete or latent SLE.

Prednisolone therapy was initiated at 15 mg/day and was subsequently increased to 30 mg/day. Erythema multiforme was alleviated quickly; but fever, polyarthritis and angioneurotic edema persisted and were ameliorated only after prednisolone was increased to 60 mg/day. We prescribed famotidine (10 mg, 2 tablets, P.O., b.i.d.) to prevent gastric ulcer. The patient's serum C3 rose to 50 mg/dL after prednisolone was increased to 60 mg/day.

Discussion

SLE, one of the collagen diseases, often develops between the third and fifth decades of life. Because this patient exhibited only three of the 11 diagnostic criteria* for SLE, a diagnosis of SLE was precluded. Instead, we made the diagnosis of SLE-related syndrome and subnamed it the Agnello-Oishi syndrome. This syndrome is characterized by erythema multiforme, angioneurotic edema, marked hypocomplementemia, and C1q precipitins of the low molecular weight type.

After the patient's intake of high-dose prednisolone, the C3 increased by 150% in spite of the immunosuppressive activity of this medication. This phenomenon gives rise to the view that an immune mechanism itself is involved in the marked hypocomplementemia associated with this particular SLE-related syndrome. Since C1q precipitins of the low molecular weight type are known to consume complement, we propose that C1q precipitins are not a result of this syndrome but a cause. Complement deficiency appears to predispose the patients to an SLE-like syndrome and may pose a high risk of progression to full-blown SLE.

involved in (= responsible for): …の原因である, …に関与する

predispose: 素因を与える, 罹患しやすくする

Lecture

-ectomy / -tomy / -stomy

Appendectomy の和訳は「虫垂切除術」である。–tomy は切開術（切断術），–stomy は造瘻術（フィステル形成術），–ectomy は切除術（摘出術）を意味する。enterotomy は「腸切開術」，enterostomy は「腸造瘻術」，enterectomy は「腸切除術」である。

line 12

Visual acuity: 視力の表記

視力は米国では"20/50"のように表記するのが普通であるが，日本では"0.4"のように表記する。米国での視力 20/20 は日本での視力 1.0 と同じであり，米国での視力を割り算すれば日本での視力になる。

lines 26–28

Prescriptions: 処方箋の書き方

line 63

　米国と日本では処方箋の書き方が異なるので注意を要する。米国では「1回〇錠を1日〇回投与」という書き方をするが，日本では1日量を書き，「〇回に分服」という指示をするのが普通である。

　米国ではオーダーシート等に "famotidine 10 mg, 2 tablets, P.O., b.i.d." のような指示を書くことが多いが，これは「ファモチジン 10 mg 錠を1回2錠，経口で1日2回投与する」という意味であり，1日の投与量は 40 mg になる。これを「ファモチジン 10 mg 錠を2錠，経口で1日2回」と和訳すると，日本人は「1日量が2錠で2回に分服」と解釈してしまい，1日の投与量が 20 mg と誤解してしまう。

　「1日 20 mg，2回に分服」を英訳すると，"a dosage of 20 mg/day in two divided doses" になる。dosage は用量，dose は1回量である。

　P.O. とか b.i.d. という略語は米国では広く使われているので，覚えておく必要がある。

Third decade の和訳

line 70

　Third decade は 30 歳代ではなく，20 歳代である。0～9 歳が first decade であり，second decade は 10 歳代である。30 歳代は fourth decade または 30s であり，third decade ではない。

Percent of increase: 〇％増加

line 79

　Increased **by** 150% は「150%だけ増加した」という意味であり，「150%に増加した」は increased **to** 150% である。Serum C3 は 20 mg/dL であったのが 50 mg/dL になったので，20 mg/dL を 100% とすると 150％だけ増加して 250% になったことになる。

Exercises

1. **Comprehension**

    Write one complete answer on each line.

    1. According to this patient's medical history, the period from onset of symptoms to recent hospitalization was _____ .

        about thirty years

        about three months

        about two years

        about six years

    2. By what route did the patient take famotidine?

        _____

        She took it by subcutaneous injection.

        She took it by mouth.

        She took it by intramuscular injection.

        She took it by intravenous infusion.

    3. How much famotidine did the patient take per day?

        _____

        She took 10 milligrams a day

        She took 20 milligrams a day.

        She took 30 milligrams a day.

        She took 40 milligrams a day.

2. Reasoning

Write A, B, C, or D (one answer each). The answer must fit the sentence grammatically and logically.

1. To qualify for publication in a medical journal, every case report must exhibit something unusual. The unusual aspect of this case was that ____ .

    A. the patient had Raynaud's phenomenon and sclerodactylia
    B. the patient had undergone an appendectomy
    C. the patient had marked hypocomplementemia and C1q precipitins of the low molecular weight type
    D. the members of the patient's immediate family did not have the same syndrome

2. Why did the doctors prescribe famotidine? _____

    A. They prescribed famotidine because the stomach cannot develop an ulcer.
    B. They prescribed famotidine because famotidine suppresses C1q precipitins of the low molecular weight type.
    C. They prescribed famotidine because famotidine enhances the efficacy of the steroid medication.
    D. They prescribed famotidine to protect the stomach from developing an ulcer as a side-effect of the steroid.

3. It is generally understood that ____ .

    A. prednisolone stimulates, or increases, one's immune activity
    B. prednisolone suppresses, or reduces, one's immune activity
    C. prednisolone has no effect on one's immune activity
    D. prednisolone is a biological marker, or indicator, of hypocomplementemia

4. The author of this case report believes that _____ .

   A. C1q precipitins cause hypocomplementemia
   B. erythema multiforme produces C1q precipitins
   C. hypocomplementemia causes precipitation of C1q
   D. hypocomplementemia controls the immune activity

5. As seen in the author's conclusion, the main instructive value of this case report is related to _____ .

   A. history of the syndrome
   B. treatment of the syndrome
   C. life expectancy of the patient
   D. pathogenesis of the syndrome

3. **Structure of the Case Report**

   Number these components from 1 to 7, in the order of their appearance in this case report.

   _____ Treatment

   _____ Diagnosis

   _____ The patient's medical history

   _____ X-ray and routine blood chemical tests

   _____ Physical examination

   _____ The patient's presenting complaint

   _____ Hematologic and immunologic laboratory tests

4. **Using Rx Symbols and Abbreviations**

   In Table 11-1, write the English meaning on the line at the right. A few are filled in.

   Table 11-1.   Terminology used when prescribing medications.

Rx Abbreviation	Meaning in Latin		Meaning in English
a.c., A.C., ac	*ante cibum*	食前に	_____
ad lib.	*ad libitum*	適宜に	as desired, given freely
b.i.d., B.I.D., bid	*bis in die*	1日2回	_____
gtt., gtt	*gutta*	滴	_____
h.s., hs	*hora somni*	就寝前に	_____
M.	*misce*	混和せよ	mix
N.P.O., NPO	*nil per os*	絶食	nothing by mouth
p.c., P.C., pc	*post cibum*	食後に	_____
P.O., PO, po	*per os*	経口で	_____
p.r.n., PRN, prn	*pro re nata*	必要に応じて	as needed
q.d., qd	*quaque die*	毎日	_____
q.4 h., q4h	*quaque 4 hora*	4時間毎に	_____
q.6 h., q6h	*quaque 6 hora*	6時間毎に	every six hours
q.i.d., qid	*quater in die*	1日4回	_____
scmel in d.	*semel in die*	1日1回	_____
Sig.	*signa*	表示せよ	label, sign (instructions on how to use the medicine, written on the label of the container)
stat., STAT	*statim*	直ちに	immediately
t.i.d., T.i.d., tid	*ter in die*	1日3回	_____

In addition, See Table 9-2 (p. 93)

5. **Comprehension**

Circle the one correct answer for each question below. 例: A. Ⓑ

1. 視力 20/40 はどちらか。

    A. 0.5　　　　　　　　　　　B. 2.0

2. phenytoin sodium 100 mg, 2 capsules, P.O., b.i.d. の 1 日投与量はどちらか。

    A. 200 mg　　　　　　　　　B. 400 mg

3. a dosage of 30 mg, in three divided doses の意味はどちらか。

    A. 1 日 30 mg，3 回に分服　　B. 1 回 30 mg，1 日 3 回

4. fifth decade はどちらか。

    A. 50 歳代　　　　　　　　　B. 40 歳代

5. increased to 110% の意味はどちらか。

    A. 110%に増加した　　　　　B. 110%だけ増加した

6. decreased by 20% の意味はどちらか。

    A. 20%に減少した　　　　　B. 20%だけ減少した

7. SLE の診断基準に入っているのはどちらか。

    A. hepatic disorder　　　　　B. photosensitivity

8. Agnello–Oishi syndrome の別名はどちらか。

    A. SLE with marked hypocomplementemia　　B. SLE-related syndrome

Lecture

Why are 4 criteria necessary for a diagnosis of SLE?

The American College of Rheumatology (ACR) によると，狼瘡様症候群 (a lupus-like syndrome，不完全あるいは潜在性狼瘡) 患者の 3 分の 1 しか本格的な SLE にならないとみられている．したがって，このような患者も含めた予後についての研究がなされた場合，SLE 患者の予後に関する記載は実際の予後より良い，誤ったものになり，治療の目的や患者のための管理過程を妨げる可能性がある．

3 分の 1; one-third

Table 11–2. Classification criteria for systemic lupus erythematosus, provided by the American College of Rheumatology (1997).*

Criterion 基準項目	Condition as Required for a Diagnosis of SLE SLE の診断に必要な条件
1. Malar rash 頬部紅斑	Fixed erythema on the cheeks 頬にみられる固定性の紅斑
2. Discoid rash 円板状皮疹	Erythematous raised patches on the skin 皮膚にみられる隆起性紅斑
3. Photosensitivity 光線過敏症	Skin rash resulting from unusual reaction to sunlight 日光に異常反応した結果みられる皮疹
4. Oral ulcers 口腔内潰瘍	Oral or nasopharyngeal ulceration, usually painless 無痛性の口腔・鼻咽頭潰瘍
5. Arthritis 関節炎	Involving two or more peripheral joints 2 ヵ所以上の末梢関節炎
6. Serositis 漿膜炎	Either pleuritis or pericarditis 胸膜炎または心膜炎
7. Renal disorder 腎障害	Either persistent proteinuria >0.5 g/day or cellular casts 0.5g/日以上の持続性蛋白尿，または細胞性円柱
8. Neurologic disorder 神経障害	Either seizures or psychosis in the absence of offending drugs 原因薬物がない状態での痙攣または精神病
9. Hematologic disorder 血液異常	Hemolytic anemia, leukopenia, lymphopenia, or thrombopenia 溶血性貧血，白血球減少，リンパ球減少，または血小板減少
10. Immunologic disorder 免疫異常	Anti-dsDNA antibody, anti-Sm antibody, or antiphospholipid antibody 抗二本鎖 DNA 抗体陽性，抗 Sm 抗体陽性，または抗リン脂質抗体陽性
11. Antinuclear antibodies (ANA) 抗核抗体	An abnormal titer of ANA by immunofluorescence or equivalent assay　免疫蛍光法もしくは同等の方法で検出可能な抗核抗体の異常高値

* The diagnosis of systemic lupus erythematosus requires the presence of 4 or more of these 11 classification criteria, serially or simultaneously, during any period of observation.
観察中にこれら 11 項目の症状のうち 4 つ以上が連続的，または同時に出現することが SLE の診断を下す基準となる．

Exercise

6. Diagnostic Criteria

Of the 11 diagnostic criteria, which three did this patient have? On each line below, write one criterion in English, and put the corresponding number from Table 11–2 (p. 119).

No.   Criterion

_____   _____

_____   _____

_____   _____

For Further Study

I heard that foreign universities do not use ○ and ×. Is that true?

英語圏の国では，○や×の印は使いません。通常使われるのは以下の4つです。

- circle the answer [例: (A.)   B.]
- write the answer beside the question [例: 1. _A_ , 2. ___]
- check, or tick, the correct answer
  [例: _✓_ Male, ___ Female]
- make an x beside the correct answer
  [例: ___ Male, _X_ Female]

海外に留学した場合，「間違い」のつもりで×を書くと，それが「正しい」と解釈されてしまいます。○に関しても，○はゼロの意味でしかないという国が多く，間違いの素になるので注意してください。

What is the difference between an oral case report and a published case report?

　医学雑誌に載っているような症例（published case report）は患者に現われている症状で始まりますが，口頭での症例提示（oral case report）は通常，疾患名を述べることから始まります。指導医，インターン，時には医学生もが，日常的にお互いに口頭での症例提示をします。少人数でコーヒーを飲みながらだったり，病院のすべての専門分野の医師が集まる回診（grand rounds）のときだったり，あるいは週に1，2回行われる指導医による回診のとき（attending rounds）や毎朝行われる引継ぎのとき（working rounds）などに行います。救急外来での症例提示の場合以外は，症例の背景についてまず述べはじめるか，あるいは単に「○○の特異な症例について報告します」（"Today we report an unusual case of …"）などのように話しはじめることもあります。

Checkpoint　When to say "case," when to say "patient"

　"Case"と"patient"は使い分けが必要です。例えばunusual（特異な）のは「患者」ではなく「症例」です。また，"Case"は人ではないので生まれたり亡くなったりしません。"This case died three weeks after admission"という表現は避け，"This patient（または person, man, woman, child) died three weeks after admission"を使います。症例報告は統計的な事柄の報告ではなく，患者（人）の報告だからです。また，caseは関係代名詞にwhichをとり，patientはwhoをとります。

COLUMN

Specializing

● **What is "board certification"?** *

　米国では研修期間（residency）終了後，専門医の試験を受けるのが通例です．認定試験のなかには1，2名の指導医が症例を提示し，受験者の知識や経験を問う難しい質問を浴びせるものもあります．American College of Rheumatology（ACR）ではSLEを含むリウマチ病学の認定試験を行い，合格した医師はACRの専門医の資格が得られます．専門医の認定資格は医療を行うのに必ず必要というわけではありませんが，もっていればより高い評価が得られますし，おそらく収入も高くなります．医学のどの分野でもそれぞれの専門医認定機関があります．
（上記のように，米国では専門医学会の名前に"College"または"Board"を使い，イギリスでは"Society"を使います．）

● **Can a Japanese doctor be a member of the ACR?**

　現在，American College of Rheumatologyには世界中から臨床医，研究者，看護師，理学療法士，作業療法士，心理学者，ソーシャルワーカーなどが会員になっています．日本人会員の名簿は下記のホームページを参照して下さい：

〈http://www.rheumatology.org〉

* Between October, 2005, and the next few years, a number of Boards are revising their certification requirements. Up-to-date information can be found at the American Board of Medical Specialties home page < www.abms.org >.

● **Do those doctors have to take tests every few years?**

　学会員は7年から10年に1回，再認定を受けなければ，その分野の専門医として医療を行う資格を失うとなっている学会がほとんどです。

　米国では，専門の認定医であろうとなかろうと，医師は皆，毎年 Continuing Medical Education（CME）が課せられています。医学雑誌に掲載されているテストに答えたり，医学会や講演会に参加したり，またビデオでの講習などを受けることで1年に50単位程度を取ることができます。

● **Can we take a look at a sample test?**

　主な医学雑誌の最後には，ほとんど毎号に質問が掲載されています。例えば The *New England Journal of Medicine* 誌では各号の中から3つほど論文を取りあげ，その論文に関する重要な質問が2つから4つ，多肢選択式で答えるようになっています。指示文はそれぞれの質問の右側に書かれています。答えはコンピュータやFAXで送信できます。

Part 4: Reading the Case Report

Chapter 12 Case Report: A 53-year-old Woman with Sudden Onset of Double Vision

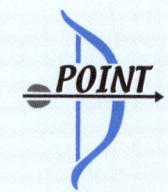

POINT
- この症例の特徴は何か。医学雑誌に掲載される価値は何か。
- この症例が医師や医学生に与える教育的メッセージは何か。

Reading

CD track 27

Case report

A 53-year-old woman presented with sudden onset of double vision and was admitted to this hospital. Her medical history was unremarkable except for hypertension, and at 16 she had had pyelonephritis. Her father died of gastric carcinoma when he was 48.

On admission, the patient's blood pressure was 180/100 mmHg. Neurological examination showed somnolence, bilateral ptosis, complete right oculomotor nerve palsy (Fig. 1), monocular downbeat nystagmus of the left eye, impairment of both adduction and upward movement of the left eye, left hemiparesis, and bilateral ataxia. Monocular downbeat nystagmus was present in the left eye, regardless of the gaze of the eye.

Laboratory examination revealed hyperlipidemia, and echocardiography showed left ventricular hypertro-

present:〔問題・状態・症状などを〕呈する

pyelonephritis: 腎盂腎炎 [pàiələnifráitis]

180/100 mmHg:〔読み方〕180 over 100 millimeters of mercury

somnolence: 傾眠

ptosis (drooping eyelid): 下垂〔症〕 [tóusis]

oculomotor nerve (= cranial nerve III): 動眼神経

palsy: 麻痺

nystagmus: 眼振

hyperlipidemia: 高脂血症

hypertrophy: 肥大

phy. Computed tomography (CT) and magnetic resonance imaging (MRI) disclosed infarction in the right midbrain and in the thalamus (Fig. 2). Right vertebral angiography indicated no venous abnormality.

Diagnosis and therapeutic intervention

Our diagnosis was brain infarction localized unilaterally in the right paramedian thalamopeduncular region. Anticoagulant therapy was initiated.

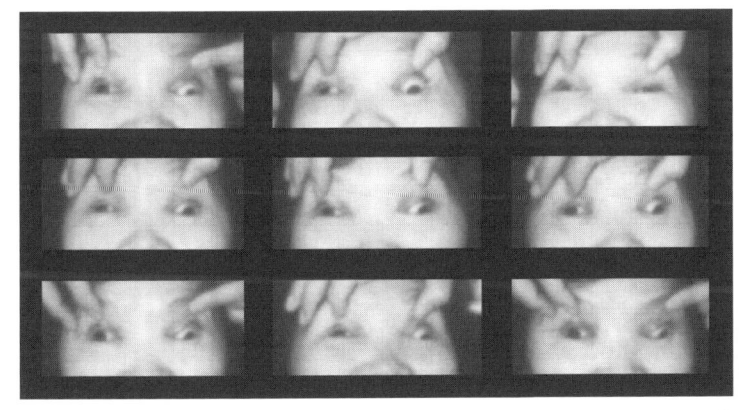

Fig. 1. Ocular movement. Photographs show severe abduction of the left eye and slight abduction of the right eye. On presentation, the patient displayed a noticeably eccentric position of the left eye, and she was unable to move the eye either upward or medially. Close examination showed that in the right eye, as well, upward movement and adduction were restricted, though this was not conspicuous at first.

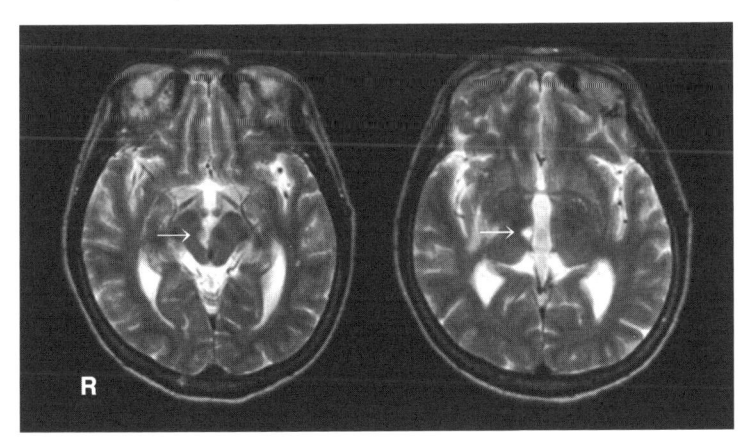

Fig. 2. Magnetic Resonance Images of the brain. A T_2-weighted image (TR 3,500 msec, TE 100 msec) shows areas of high signal (arrows) in the right midbrain and thalamus, suggesting paramedian thalamopeduncular infarction.

disclosed: 明らかにする

infarction: 梗塞

angiography: 血管造影〔法〕

paramedian: 傍正中の，正中傍の

thalamopeduncular: 視床〔大脳〕脚の

anticoagulant therapy: 抗凝固療法

ocular: 眼の

abduction: 外転

eccentric (= away from the center): 離心性の (中心から離れた方向に)

adduction: 内転

conspicuous: 顕著な

msec (= milliseconds): ミリ秒

Discussion

Monocular downbeat nystagmus is extremely rare, and the responsible lesion has not been clarified.[1–3] In the present case, the responsible site of infarction was the paramedian thalamopeduncular region, which is supplied by the superior mesencephalic and posterior thalamosubthalamic arteries.[4] Since both of these arteries branch from the same artery, i.e., the basilar artery, it is plausible that the infarctions found in the midbrain and thalamus occurred simultaneously and that occlusions in these arteries would be attributable to a common mechanism. Paramedian thalamopeduncular infarction is typified by clinical variations reflecting the topography and extent of ischemic damage,[4] with or without monocular downbeat nystagmus.[2,4] To date, two other cases have been reported in which oculomotor nerve palsy in one eye was associated with downbeat nystagmus in the other eye.[2] As in our patient, the infarctions were unilateral and limited to the paramedian thalamopeduncular region.[2]

Bilateral downbeat nystagmus is generally associated with a lesion in the cerebellum and has also been reported to result from an infarction in the midbrain.[5] Monocular downbeat nystagmus has been attributed to dysfunction of the ipsilateral brachium conjunctivum.[1] Curiously, however, in our patient as well as in the two cases reported by Jacome,[2] monocular downbeat nystagmus occurred in the eye contralateral to the midbrain lesion. The possibility cannot be ruled out that in this case the monocular downbeat nystagmus was caused by the unilateral lesions found in the central nervous system. However, taking into account all the patient's symptoms and clinical findings, we believe that bilateral downbeat nystagmus was present but masked by a concomitant pathologic disturbance. Given that oculomotor nerve palsy was present in the opposite eye, we postulate that the present case as well as the two cases reported by Jacome can be explained as bilateral downbeat nystagmus manifesting as monocular downbeat nystagmus.

A small infarction in the brainstem is often undetectable by CT scan, making clinical manifestation all the more important in establishing a diagnosis. For example, in a patient with unilateral oculomotor nerve palsy and contralateral downbeat nystagmus, a paramedian thalamopeduncular infarction is suspected even if CT scan is normal. A number of syndromes are known to involve the cranial nerves and/or brainstem, such as Weber's syndrome, Millard–Gubler syndrome, Wallenberg's syndrome, Foster Kennedy's syndrome, Vernet's syndrome, and Collet–Sicard syndrome. Knowing the manifestations of these various syndromes can be helpful in determining the site of the lesion.

masked by: 覆い隠される

concomitant (= coexisting): 付随する，伴う

Given that: 〜と仮定すると，〜なので

postulate (= speculate; conjecture): 仮定する，推測する

manifest: 現われる

References

1. Bogousslavsky J, Regili F. 1985. Monocular downbeat nystagmus. *J Neurol* 231:99–101.
2. Jacome DE. 1986. Monocular downbeat nystagmus. *Ann Ophthalmol* 18:293–296.
3. Nozaki S, Mukuno K, Ishikawa S. 1983. Internuclear ophthalmoplegia associated with ipsilateral downbeat nystagmus and contralateral incyclorotatory nystagmus. *Ophthalmologica* 187:210–216.
4. Tatemichi TK, Steinke W, Duncan C, Bell JA, Odel JG, Behrens

MM, Hilal SK, Mohr JP. 1992. Paramedian thalamopeduncular infarction: clinical syndromes and magnetic resonance imaging. *Ann Neurol* 32:162–171.

5. Yee RD. 1989. Downbeat nystagmus: characteristics and localization of lesions. *Trans Am Ophthalmol Soc* 87:984–1032.

- Oishi M, Mochizuki Y. 1996. Ipsilateral oculomotor nerve palsy and contralateral downbeat nystagmus: a syndrome caused by unilateral paramedian thalamopeduncular infarction. *J Neurol* 244: 132–133.
- 伊藤正男，他（編）：望月-大石症候群．『医学書院 医学大辞典』，医学書院，2003，p. 2428.

Exercises

1. Comprehension

Write either <u>True</u> or <u>False</u> on each line.

_____ 1. Midbrain infarction is known to cause bilateral downbeat nystagmus.

_____ 2. Bilateral downbeat nystagmus is known to cause midbrain infarction.

_____ 3. This patient may have had bilateral downbeat nystagmus, although it was not detectable.

_____ 4. In this patient, upbeat nystagmus was noticeable in one eye.

_____ 5. In this patient, downbeat nystagmus was noticeable in one eye.

_____ 6. Left unilateral nystagmus is the same as left monocular nystagmus.

_____ 7. In this patient, nystagmus was a cause, not a result.

_____ 8. In this patient, nystagmus was a result, not a cause.

_____ 9. High blood pressure in this patient may have been an early sign of eminent infarction.

_____ 10. Small infarction in the brainstem often eludes detection by CT scan.

2. **Reasoning**

    Write A, B, or C on the line.

    1. Anticoagulation therapy was initiated _____ .
        A. to restore the damaged tissue (infarct)
        B. as a palliative treatment to prevent blood clots that would likely cause further damage
        C. because the superior mesencephalic and posterior thalamosubthalamic arteries supply that region of the brain

    2. This case report forcuses mainly on _____ .
        A. treatment
        B. diagnosis
        C. prevention

    3. The unusual aspect of this case report is that _____ .
        A. double vision had occurred without warning
        B. no lesion was present in the cerebellum
        C. nystagmus occurred in the eye on the side opposite that of the midbrain lesion

4. In this figure, which combination shows the site of the presenting nystagmus that was conspicuous and easily recognized and the sites of the MRI findings in this case report? _____

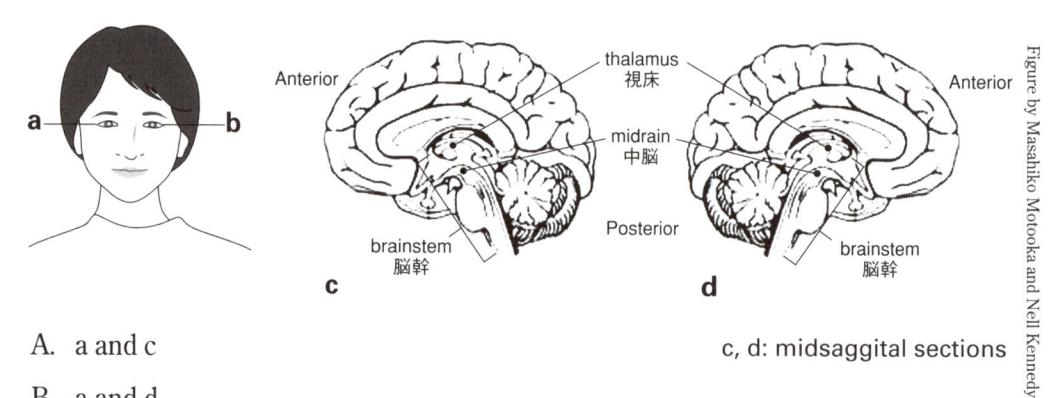

c, d: midsaggital sections

Figure by Masahiko Motooka and Nell Kennedy

A. a and c
B. a and d
C. b and c
D. b and d

3. Vocabulary

From the box, write the word that matches the general English meaning. Each is used once only.

_____	1. located higher
_____	2. pertaining to two sides
_____	3. drawing away from the midline
_____	4. located on or near the back of the body
_____	5. pertaining to one eye
_____	6. drawing toward the midline
_____	7. deviant, or not normal
_____	8. situated underneath
_____	9. pertaining to one side
_____	10. pertaining to the same side
_____	11. pertaining to the opposite side
_____	12. located on or near the front of the body

abduction
abnormal
adduction
anterior
bilateral
contralateral
inferior
ipsilateral
monocular
posterior
superior
unilateral

Lecture

What can we expect from a Case Report?

■ Key feature
　症例報告の特徴は，その症例を示すことで他の医師が同様の問題に遭遇した場合の認識や対処に役立てることです。

医師，臨床医：clinician

■ Message for the reader
　症例報告はどれもまれな症例を採り上げていますが，まれであるという理由だけで掲載されているわけではありません。どの症例報告にも読者へのメッセージが込められています。そのメッセージを読むために症例報告を読むのです。

■ Message type A
1. 同様の症例に遭遇した場合に，より迅速に診断ができるよう，そのような病状に対する認識を高めておくこと。
2. ある治療方針が他の治療法より適切かつ効果的であることを示しておくこと。

より適切な：more suitable

より効果的な：more effective

■ Message type B
1. まれな，おそらくは知られてもいない併発症状をもっていて，そのために治療において相反する2つの優先順位が生じてしまうような患者を提示すること。例えば，患者がある薬が禁忌となるような合併症をもっていて，薬物療法が逆の効果をもたらすというような不都合なことが起こった場合は，症例報告ではその見落としを隠さずに書きます。そのメッセージが明確ならば，隠さずに報告することが世界中の医師に多大な利益をもたらします。
2. まれな，あるいは特異な合併症を示している患者や，従来とは異なる治療法が必要な患者の提示。

併発症状：concomitant condition

禁忌である：contraindicated (compare p. 25 Scientific English, 1)

逆効果：adverse effect

合併症：complication

従来とは異なる治療法：unconventional therapeutic procedure

■ Chronological structure of published Case Reports

1. 今日，雑誌に掲載されるような症例報告ではほとんどがまず初めに患者の性別，年齢，現れている症状を示します。
2. 次に患者自身の病歴および肉親の病歴（家族歴）について示します。
3. 身体所見の結果，さらに血液検査，尿検査，免疫検査等の検査結果が示されます。
4. X線，CT，またはその他の画像。
5. 診断と治療法。
6. 最後に患者または疾患の経過が示されます。
7. 一流の学術誌では，その後の結果，例えば，①1年後，患者は介護なしで歩行でき，日常の生活動作も自力でできている，とか，②入院5週間後に死亡した，等の記載もあります。

　一般の医学論文と異なり，症例報告でのDiscussionは他の論文を引用して述べるような長いものではなく，通常はごく簡単なものです。症例報告のDiscussionの主な目的は，医師の決断がどのようになされたかの説明と，そこから学ぶべき点は何かを示すことです。

■ Do Case Reports count as research?

　はい。以前は症例報告は研究とみなされなかったため編集者もあまり興味を示しませんでしたが，今日では一流の学術誌はほとんど毎号で症例報告を掲載しています。なかにはその症例を担当した医師たちの詳しい会話の内容まで載せているものもあります。通常，症例は実際の診療に直接関連しますので，一般の医師にとって学術誌が実際的な有効性をもつために症例報告が一役買っているのです。

ほとんど：almost all

現れている症状：complaint (presenting symptoms)

病歴：medical history

肉親：immediate family

身体所見：physical examination

血液〔学的〕検査：hematological (hematologic) test

尿検査：urinalysis

X線：X-ray

CT（コンピュータ断層撮影）：computed tomography

結果：outcome

日常生活動作：activities of daily living (ADL)

入院：admission

研究：research

一流の学術誌：prestigious journals

…に直接関連する：have direct bearing on

実際的な有効性：practical relevance

Exercise

4. **The Case Report in Medical Journals**

   1. **Which one of these statements is NOT true? Put an X beside A–E to indicate your answer.**

      A. The case report is usually about a rare condition.

      B. The case report usually describes the clinical signs of a patient's condition.

      C. The case report may provide an early warning system of a new and emerging disease.

      D. The case report provides strong evidence for the cause of a condition.

      E. The case report often contains atypical descriptions.

   2. **Which of these statements are true? Circle A–E to indicate your answers.**

      A. The case report is about a single patient.

      B. The case report is a collection of several cases of patients being treated for the same condition.

      C. The purpose of the case report is to present a particular history, clinical description, diagnosis, treatment and/or prognosis to the medical profession.

      D. In the absence of other sources of information, the case report helps the physicians to acquire clinical evidence.

      E. All of the above.

Lecture

「死亡する」という場合の前置詞

病気で死亡する場合は"die of," 事故などがもとで死亡する場合は"die from," 戦闘で死亡する場合は"die in battle" です。

Two or more と more than two

Two or more は2を含み，more than two は2を含みません。「2以上」は2を含むので "two or more" です。同様に three or fewer (three or less) は3以下で，fewer than three (less than three) は3未満です。

人名の発音

日本の医学書や医学辞典をみると，例えばフランス人の人名をフランス語読みではなく，ローマ字読みまたは英語読みでカタカナ表記しているものがたくさんあります。しかし，本来人名はその人の母国語読みで発音すべきものなので，正しい発音を覚えてください。

また，人名のハイフンについては次のことを知っておいてください。例えば，Foster Kennedy's syndrome (1人の姓と名) ではハイフンを入れず，Millard–Gubler syndrome (2人の姓) ではハイフンを入れます。また，Brown–Séquard's syndrome (1人の姓) は最初からハイフンが入っている姓です。ちなみに，é のような´印(アクサン・テギュ)は，強く発音するという意味ではありません。

Exercises

5. Precision of expression

Circle the one correct answer for each question below. 例: A. Ⓑ

1. 「過労がもとで死亡した」はどちらか。

    A. died of overwork   B. died from overwork

2. 「心筋梗塞で死亡した」はどちらか。

    A. died of myocardial infarction   B. died from myocardial infarction

3. 血圧 120/80 mmHg の読み方はどちらか。

    A. 120 per 80   B. 120 over 80

4. ileostomy はどちらか。(see p. 112)

    A. 回腸造瘻術   B. 回腸切開術

5. under 18 years of age (younger than 18) はどちらか。

    A. 18歳以下   B. 18歳未満

6. lidocaine は局所麻酔薬や不整脈の治療薬として用いられているが，国際的に lidocaine の読み方はどちらか。

    A. リドカイン   B. ライダケイン

7. more than one limb はどちらか。

    A. 1肢以上   B. 2肢以上

6. Vocabulary

From the box, choose one expression each. Write A–T on the line. All answers are used one time each.

____ 1. Fast left-to-right movement, or fluttering, of the eyeball

____ 2. Fast up-and-down movement, or fluttering, of the eyeball

____ 3. Drooping eyelid

____ 4. Outside the eyeball. The patient complained of pain inside the eye, but the cause was _____ . A small nodule had formed in the upper eyelid; but when the nodule was removed, the pain inside the eye was eliminated.

____ 5. Out of the center.

____ 6. Slight paralysis affecting one side of the body.

____ 7. Loss of coordination of the muscles, especially in the extremities

____ 8. Sleepiness, drowsiness

____ 9. High blood pressure

____ 10. Enlargement

____ 11. Happening at the same time

____ 12. A sign of an illness

____ 13. Present together with another

____ 14. To show plainly, to display symptoms

____ 15. To propose an idea, to assume, to guess

____ 16. Believable, reasonable

____ 17. Said to be caused by

____ 18. To come to the hospital for examination or treatment

____ 19. Without anything especially unusual

____ 20. To make clear, to make known for sure

A. ataxia
B. attributable to
C. clarify
D. concomitant
E. eccentric
F. extraocular
G. hemiparesis
H. horizontal nystagmus
I. hypertension
J. hypertrophy
K. manifest
L. plausible
M. postulate
N. present
O. ptosis
P. simultaneously
Q. somnolence
R. symptom
S. unremarkable
T. vertical nystagmus

Appendix

Training to Listen like a Scientist
In search of clinical evidence　臨床的根拠の探求　　CD track 9

1. **Q. Do medical journals use information from the Voice of America and National Public Radio?**

   A. No, because the VOA and NPR did not do the research. Their main service is to announce important medical news quickly in simple words that anybody can understand.
   いいえ。VOAやNPRが研究をしたわけではありません。放送局の主な業務は、だれにでもわかる簡潔な言葉で、迅速に重要な医療ニュースを伝えることです。

2. **Q. Is the original research paper the same as the VOA and NPR news report?**

   A. The main information is the same, but the news reports are much shorter and <u>the data are usually rounded</u> to help the listeners pick up the main points quickly. In the study on diuretics for treating high blood pressure (Chapter 4), the VOA says, "<u>More than 42,000</u> people in <u>more than 600 hospitals</u> took part." But the full study involved <u>a total of 33,357 participants</u> from <u>623 hospitals</u>. (See 3 below.)
   主な情報は同じですが、ニュースのレポートはかなり短く、<u>データは通常、端数を省略して大まかな数字にされます</u>。これは視聴者が要点を素早く汲み取ることができるためにです。例えば、Chapter 4の高血圧の治療に利尿薬を使用するという<u>研究で、VOAは「600以上の病院</u>の42,000人以上が参加した」とレポートしています<u>が、研究全体では623の病院からの合計33,357人</u>が関わっています。（次頁3を参照）

3. **Q. Why is there such a difference?**

   A. For one thing, VOA took the total number of hypertensive patients who were <u>screened for eligibility to participate in the study</u>. Second, <u>the study criteria</u> were not just patients with hypertension, but patients with hypertension <u>plus</u> at least one other risk factor of coronary heart disease (CHD). Almost 9,000 hypertensive candidates were excluded from the study (a) because they were not at high risk for CHD; (b) because some died before the study treatments began; (c) because their conditions were too risky for them to change their medications; or (d) because some had other coexisting diseases that required separate treatment. Nevertheless, the VOA report was right about the fact that this was the largest study on high blood pressure treatment ever carried out in the United States.

一つに，VOAはこの研究へ参加資格があるとして選ばれた，高血圧患者の全体数を数えています。第2に，研究の基準は，単に高血圧の患者というだけでなく，高血圧に加えて，冠状動脈性心疾患（CHD）の危険因子を少なくとももう一つ別にもっている患者でした。高血圧を患う参加候補者約9,000人は，(a) CHDの危険性が高くない，(b) この研究による治療が始まる前に死亡した，(c) 治療薬を替えるには体調があまりにも危険であることが判明した，(d) 別な治療を必要とする他の疾患を抱えていた，などの理由で研究から除外されました。しかし，これがこれまでアメリカ合衆国で行われた高血圧の治療に関する研究で最大規模であるという点で，VOAのレポートは正しいものです。

4. Q. Why did the original research paper report so many patients if some did not complete the study?

A. To show that they were not manipulating the data to support their own private ideas (bias), researchers must tell exactly how many patients dropped out before or during the study, why each one dropped out, and whether any data from the dropouts were in the final analyses. By being transparent and honest, medical research has earned respect and trust as Evidence-Based Medicine. 独自の見解を支えるためにデータを操作したわけではないことを示すために，研究の前，研究の最中に患者が何人抜けたか，なぜ抜けたか，途中で抜けた患者のデータを最終的な分析で数えているかを研究者は正確に告げなければなりません。このような透明性と誠実さがあって初めて医学研究は根拠に基づいた医療（EBM）としての敬意と信頼を得てきたのです。

5. Q. Were there any other differences between the VOA report and the original research on diuretics?

A. (1) VOA said the average age of the patients was 67 years, which is true. The original paper adds that they were 55 years old or older. (2) The research paper tells the **names** of the medicines tested: the calcium channel blocker was <u>amlodipine</u>; the ACE inhibitor was <u>lisinopril</u>; and the diuretic was <u>chlorthalidone</u>.

（1）VOAは患者の平均年齢を67歳としていますが，間違いありません。元になった論文では，患者が55歳以上であったと説明しています。（2）元の論文では，試験に使われた薬の名称に触れています。カルシウムチャネル遮断薬がアムロジピン，ACE阻害薬がリジノプリル，利尿薬がクロルタリドンです。

6. Q. **Where can we find the original research paper?**

   A. Probably in the university library. Here are the title and source:

   おそらく，大学の図書館にあります。論文のタイトルと出典は以下の通りです。

   ALLHAT Officers and Coordinators for the ALLHAT Collaborative Research Group. The Antihypertensive and Lipid-Lowering Treatment to Prevent Heart Attack Trial: Major outcomes in high-risk hypertensive patients randomized to angiotensin-converting enzyme inhibitor or calcium channel blocker vs diuretic. 2002. *JAMA* 288 (23): 2981–2997.

7. Q. **Does the VOA report exaggerate?**

   A. No. The VOA journalists are highly respected for reliable reporting around the world. However, unless we <u>train ourselves to listen like a scientist</u>, we could get the idea that ALL diuretics work better than those other drugs in the study. <u>This research did not test ALL diuretics</u>. The study published in the *Journal of the American Medical Association (JAMA)* involved <u>one type of diuretic</u>, and the conclusion was specifically that the <u>thiazide-type diuretics</u> are superior in preventing one or more major forms of coronary vascular disease and that they should be preferred for <u>first-step</u> antihypertensive therapy.

   いいえ。VOAの記者は信頼できる報道をすることで世界中で高く評価されています。しかし，<u>科学者としての聴き方ができるように訓練</u>しなければ，すべての利尿薬がよく効いて，研究で使用された薬よりも優れていると考える視聴者がいるかもしれません。<u>この研究ではすべての利尿薬を試験した訳ではありません</u>。アメリカ医学学会誌（*JAMA*）で発表された研究では，<u>一つのタイプの薬</u>が使われていて，結論は，<u>サイアザイド系利尿薬が冠動脈疾患の主な病状を1つ以上予防するのに優れていること，抗高血圧治療の<u>第一歩</u>として優先すべきことを特に述べています。

Index

A

a.c., A.C., ac (ante cibum)   117
abduction 125
absorption 69
ACE inhibitor 38
activities of daily living (ADL)
  132
ad lib. (ad libitum) 117
adduction 125
adhere 20
adjuvant therapy 20
admission 132
advance 20
adverse effect 131
afferent 20
AIDS 40
allergy 40
alleviate 94
allow ⋯ to ∼ 15
almost all 132
ambiguity 21
anecdotal experience 96
angiography 125
angioneurotic 109
ante cibum 117
antecubital 79
antibiotic 2
antibody 43, 47, 50
antibody response 43
anticoagulant therapy 125
anti-inflammatory 24
antinuclear antibody (ANA)
  .... 110, 119
appendectomy 109, 112
arthritis 119

B

as much as 24
at bay 5
atherosclerosis 22
attack 2
(be) attenuated 87
attributable to ⋯ 69
augment 95
autosomal recessive error .. 68
azathioprine 50

b.i.d., B.I.D., bid (bis in die) 117
bacterial infection 2
barometric pressure 14
basic research 55
best bet, the 22, 25
bilateral 109
biochemical 23
biofeedback 5
biopsy 78
bis in die 117
bladder 34
blood 40
blood clot 40
blood sugar 50
blood vessel 12, 34
bloodborne 95
(be) blunted 86
brachium conjunctivum ... 126
bulge 12
bypass 22

C

C1q precipitins 110
calcium channel blocker ... 38
cancer 40
cardiac muscle 24
case 121
casts 109
cause ⋯ to ∼ 15
cell 23
cellular 23
centrifuge 80
cervical 109
chances are that ⋯ 4
cholesterol 25, 40
chronic 23, 50
clarify 126
clinician 131
clog 22
clot 23
cluster headache 2
coexisting 127
collaborator 50
compensate 69
complaint 132
complement 110
complication 40, 47, 131
computed tomography (CT)
  132
concomitant 127
concomitant condition 131
congestive heart failure 24
conjecture 127
conjunctival injection 109
conspicuous 125
contraindicated 25, 96, 131
contralateral 126
cornstarch 105
coronary artery 23

costly 34
cramps 68
cranial nerve 20
cranial nerve V 13
creatine supplementation .. 94
crossover 81
curb 23
curtail 96
cyclosporine 50

D

dampen 24
Darwinian evolution 43
debilitating 3
decade 113
deceased 32
deleterious 23
depend on the route of
    administration 69
detritus 23
diabetes mellitus 47, 96
diabetics 50
diagnose 50
diagnosis 55
diet 40
digestion 40
disaccharide 70
disclosed 125
discoid rash 119
diseased 32
disorder 3, 68
distal 109
diuretics 34, 38
dose 50
dose-response effect 79
double-blind 80
drag 32
drip 40
drug 32, 40

drug abuse 34
dura mater 12

E

eccentric 125
edema 109, 111
efferent 21
elicit 96
embed 12
ensue 23
enterectomy 112
enterostomy 112
enterotomy 112
enzyme 68
episode 2
eponym 60
ergometer 79
erythema multiforme ... 109
evolve 43
excretion 23
exercise tolerance 56, 69
expenditure 96
experiment 34
extramuscular 69

F

famotidine 113
fat 25, 47
fatty acid 25
fatty deposit 25
fatty plaque 25
ferry 13
fibrous 12
figure out 24
flexor surfaces 109
flood ··· with ∼ 13
fluorescent light 3
fructose 70

G

generator 13
genetic 22
genetic material 43
genetically engineered 50
germ 43
get one's second wind 69
given that 127
glucose 47, 69
glycogen 68
glycogen storage disease
    type V 65
glycogenolysis 58, 69
graft 22
gtt., gtt (gutta) 117

H

h.s., hs (hora somni) 117
hart 32
have direct bearing on 132
heart 32
heart attack 38
heart disease 34, 38, 40
heart failure 38
heart trouble 38
heartbeat 32
hematologic disorder 119
hematologic (hematological)
    test 132
hemolytic anemia 119
high blood pressure 23, 34, 38
HIV 43
hora somni 117
hormone 14
human-genome 22
hyperinsulinemia 87
hyperlipidemia 124
hypertrophy 124
hypothesize 58

I

i.e. 20, 126
imaging technique 12
immediate family 132
immune 40, 47
immune response 50
immune suppressive drug .. 50
immune system 43, 50
immunofluorescence 119
immunologic disorder 119
in line with 87
in vitro 95
increase 113
incubation 40
induce 95
infarction 125
infection 40, 43, 50
inflame 23
inflammation 23, 40
influenza 40
informed consent 83
ingest 96
ingested 86
ingestion 70
inhibitor 56
injection 40, 50
injest 58
insulin 47, 50
insulin-dependent diabetes 56
insulin-secreting cell 50
intact 95
interphalangeal 109
intravenous infusion 69
intravenously 3
invasion 40
involved in 112
ipsilateral 126
ischemic 126

J

Journal of the American Medical Association, the   38
juvenile diabetes 47, 50
Juvenile Diabetes Research Foundation, the 50

K

kidney disease 50

L

lacrimal 20
lactate 80
latent 111
lesion 126
leukopenia 119
lifestyle 47
lipids 25
liquid 38
liver 23, 47
loading 96
lymphadenitis 111
lymphocyte 40
lymphopenia 119

M

M. (misce) 117
malar rash 119
mandibular 21
mandibular nerve 20
manifest 127
marked 87
masked by 127
maxillary nerve 20
McArdle's disease 58
medical history 132
medical research paper 58
medication 3
meditation 4

Medline 65
mesencephalic 126
metabolism 40, 58, 68
metastasis 40
migraine 3
migraineur 4
misce 117
modest 50
more suitable 131
more effective 131
muscle glycogen phosphorylase deficiency 65
mutate 43
mutation 40, 43
myoglobinuria 68
myophosphorylase 68, 78

N

N.P.O., NPO (nil per os) .. 117
namely 20, 126
nasal 20
National Heart, Lung and Blood Institute, the 38
nausea 3
nephropathy 47
nerve 12
nerve ending 12
neurologic disorder 119
neutralizing antibody 43
New England Journal of Medicine, the 50
nil per os 117
nitric oxide (NO) 57
non-insulin-dependent diabetes
 57
nonpharmacological 4
nystagmus 124

O

obesity 40
(be) obliterated 86
occult blood 109
ocular 125
oculomotor nerve 124
on a daily basis 3
onset, the 95
ophthalmic nerve 20
oral ulcers 119
order 38
outcome 132

P

p.c., P.C., pc (post cibum) 117
P.O., PO, po (per os) 117
p.r.n., PRN, prn (pro re nata)
.... 117
paired *t*-test 80
palsy 124
pancreas 47, 50
paradoxically 24
paramedian 125
particle 43
pathophysiology 55
patient 121
peak oxidative capacity 69
pediatric 56
per os 117
perceived exertion .. 69, 79, 86
pericarditis 119
persistent 14
pharmaceutical treatment .. 22
phospholipid 25
photosensitivity 119
physical examination 132
phytohemagglutinin (PHA) 110
pill 38
placebo-controlled 81

plague 32
plaque 22, 32
platelet 40
pleuritis 119
plumbling problem 22
polyarthralgia 108
polyarthritis 109
pons 20
post cibum 117
postulate 127
practical relevance 132
preclude 111
predispose 112
prednisone 50
predominantly 58
pregnant 55
preliminary 50
prescribe 2, 111
prescriptions 113
present 124
presenting symptoms 132
prestigious journals 132
prevalence 68
prevent 38
prevention 55
primary 2
prime 13
pro re nata 117
progeny 43
progress 38
proliferation 40
prominent 12
prone to 14, 70, 97
prophylaxis 43
protein 13
proteinuria 119
protocol 79
provoke 94
proximal 109

psychosis 119
ptosis 124
P-value 80, 83
pyelonephritis 124
pyruvate 80

Q

q.4h, q4h (quaque 4 hora) 117
q.6h, q6h (quaque 6 hora) 117
q.d., qd (quaque die) 117
q.i.d., qid (quater in die) .. 117
quick fix 3

R

randomized 81
Raynaud's phenomenon .. 109
relay 20
rely on 22
remission 40
renal disorder 119
replicate 43
research 132
residency 122
residual 78
resolve 109
respiration 40
responsible 112, 126
rupture 23

S

saturated fat 24, 25
scab 23
scalp 20
sclerodactylia 109
± SE 80
sear 3
seasoned readers 58
second-wind phenomenon 69
seizure 119

selective force 43
selective pressure 43
self-contained 2, 7
self-limited 2, 7
semel in d. (semel in die) 117
sensitivity 3
sensory 13
serositis 119
shimmering light 13
shot 50
siblings 109
side effect 47
Sig. (signa) 117
single-blind 80
single-blind, randomized,
  placebo-controlled crossover
  study 70
so far 126
sodium 38
somnolence 124
speculate 127
spin; spun 80
stack of 14
staining 78
stat., STAT (statim) 117
statins 23
stem from 13
stimuli; stimulus 13
strain 43
stroke 34, 38
subsequent 96
substantial 96
sucrose 58, 70
suggest 15
surgery 22
susceptible to 95
swear by 4
swell; swollen 13
sympathetic nerve 40

symptoms 94
systemic lupus erythematosus
  (SLE) 111

T

t.i.d., T.i.d., tid (ter in die) 117
tailor … to ∼ 22
tension 2
ter in die 117
thalamopeduncular 125
thalamosubthalamic 126
that is 20, 126
third decade 111, 113
threshold 14, 96
throbbing 3
thrombopenia 119
tissue 40
to date 126
tolerance 40
topography 126
translated 94
treatment 55
trigeminal ganglion 20
trigeminal nerve 13, 20
trigger 3
(be) triggered by 78
triglyceride 25
tumor 40, 50
type 1 diabetes 50, 56
type 2 diabetes 57

U

umbrella sentence 6
unconventional therapeutic procedure 131
United States Food and Drug
  Administration, the 38
unusual 121
urinalysis 132

urine 38
urology 34

V

vaccine 40, 43
variation 43
versus 56
virologist 43
virtually 95
virus 40
visual acuity 109, 112
vomiting 3
vs (versus) 56

W

warrant 97
waste 38
white blood cell 40

X

X-ray 132

Y

yoga 4

Z

Zucker diabetic fatty rat 57

Index

あ
あいまいさ	21
明らかにする	125, 126
アテローム性動脈硬化症	22
現われている症状	132
現われる	127
〔…を〜に〕合わせる	22

い
医学論文	58
閾値	14, 96
医師	131
移植片	22
一義的な	2
一致して	87
一流の学術誌	132
一酸化窒素	57
逸話に富んだ経験	96
遺伝子の	22
インフォームド・コンセント	83

う
うっ血性心不全	24
運動耐容能	56, 69

え
影響されやすい	95
疫病	32
X線	132
エルゴメータ	79
遠位の	109
炎症	23
——を起こす	23
遠心性の	21
遠心分離器	80
円柱	109
円板状紅斑	119

お
嘔吐	3
覆い隠される	127
おそらく	4
主に	58

か
開始	95
外転	125
回避する	22
下顎神経	20
下顎の	21
かさぶた	23
下垂〔症〕	124
仮説を立てる	58
かたまり	23
合併症	131
仮定する	127
果糖	70
〔刺激に対する〕過敏性	3
考え出す	24
感覚の	13
患者	121
冠状動脈	23
眼振	124
眼神経	20
関節炎	119
完全な	95
肝臓	23
緩和する	94

き
気圧	14
〔…に〕帰する	69
基礎研究	55
逆効果	131
逆説的に	24
吸収	69
求心性の	20
強指症	109
きょうだい	109
頬部紅斑	119
胸膜炎	119
局所解剖学	126
虚血の	126
許容範囲	14
近位の	109
筋外の	69
禁忌である	25, 96, 131
緊急治療薬	3
緊張	2
筋ホスホリラーゼ	68, 78
筋ホスホリラーゼ欠損症	65

く
薬	32
屈側面	109
グリコーゲン	68
グリコーゲン分解	58
クレアチン補充	94
クロスオーバー	81
群発性頭痛	2

け
〔…の〕傾向がある	14, 70, 97
経静脈で	3
頸〔部〕の	109
傾眠	124
痙攣	68, 119
血液異常	119
血液〔学的〕検査	132
血液媒介性の	95
結果	132
結果として起こる	23
血管	12
血管運動神経性の	109
血管造影〔法〕	125
血管を詰まらせる	22

結合腕	126
血小板減少	119
血栓	23
結膜充血	109
〔…の〕原因である	112
限界	14
元気を回復する	69
研究	132
研修期間	122
顕著な	87, 125
原発の	2

こ

高インスリン血症	87
抗炎症の	24
抗核抗体	110, 119
抗凝固療法	125
口腔内潰瘍	119
高血圧〔症〕	23
高脂血症	124
抗生物質	2
光線過敏症	119
酵素	68
〔脳・脊髄の〕硬膜	12
コレステロール	25
これまで	126
梗塞	125
コーンスターチ	105
コンピュータ断層撮影	132

さ

細菌感染	2
最善の選択	22, 25
最大酸素摂取能	69
細胞の	23
削減する	96
左右の	109
三叉神経	13, 20
三叉神経節	20

し

自覚的運動	86
自覚的運動強度	69, 79
死去した	32
刺激	13
自己限定〔性〕の	2, 7
脂質	25
事実上；実質上	95
視床〔大脳〕脚の	125
視床視床下部の	126
指節間の	109
持続的な	14
疾患	3, 68
実際的な有効性	132
脂肪	25
脂肪酸	25
従来とは異なる治療法	131
手術	22
腫脹する	13
〔…の〕準備をする	13
上顎神経	20
消散する	109
症状	94
症状の発現	2
〔…から〕生じる	13
常染色体劣性異常	68
小児〔科〕の	56
消費〔量〕	96
漿膜炎	119
静脈内注射	69
症例	121
ショ糖	58, 70
処方する	2, 111
処方箋	113
視力	109, 112
腎盂腎炎	124
心筋	24
神経	12
〔軸索の〕神経終末	12

神経障害	119
腎障害	119
心臓	32
身体所見	132
診断	55
心拍	32
心膜炎	119

す

衰弱させる	3
推測する	127
ずきんずきんとする	3
スタチン	23
すなわち	20, 126

せ

生化学の	23
生検	78
精神病	119
生体外の（で）	95
正中傍の	125
セカンドウインド現象	69
責任のある	126
摂取	70
摂取した	86
摂取する	58, 96
是認する	97
線維の	12
潜血	109
潜在性の	111
染色	78
全身性エリテマトーデス（紅斑性狼瘡）	111

そ

素因を与える	112
造影技術	12
増加(増大)させる	95
相当な	96

Index

阻害因子 56
阻害薬 56
〔〜を…に〕注ぐ 13
その後の 97

──── た ────
〜対〜 56
第5脳神経 13
代謝 58, 68
代償する 69
だいたいは 58
卓越した 12
たくさんの 14
多形性紅斑 109
多発関節痛 108
多発性関節炎 109
〔…に〕頼りきる 4
〔…に〕頼る 22
蛋白質 13
蛋白尿 119
担当した医師 132
単盲検 80
単盲検無作為化プラセボ対照
　クロスオーバー試験 70

──── ち ────
知覚の 13
ちかちか光るような自覚症状
　.......................... 13
中継する 20
虫垂切除術 109, 112
中性脂肪 25
肘前の 79
中脳の 126
調子を取り戻す 69
腸切開術 112
腸切除術 112
腸造瘻術 112
〔…に〕直接関連する 132

著明な 87
治療 55

──── つ ────
対側の 126

──── て ────
低下させる 24
〔問題・状態・症状などを〕
　呈する 124
手指（足指）硬化症 109

──── と ────
動眼神経 124
糖原貯蔵症5型 65
糖原分解 58, 69
同側の 126
糖尿病 96
頭皮 20
投薬 4
投薬経路に依存する 69
特異な 121
伴う 127

──── な ────
内転 125
涙の 20

──── に ────
肉親 132
20歳代 111
二重盲検 80
日常生活動作 132
二糖類 70
鈍らされる 86
入院 132
乳酸塩 80
尿検査 132
妊娠している 55

──── の ────
脳橋 20
脳神経 20
残りの 78

──── は ────
〔あらかじめ〕排除する ... 111
排泄 23
バイパスを形成する 22
吐気 3
運ぶ 13
白血球減少 119
鼻の 20
破裂する 23
斑 22, 32
反対側の 126

──── ひ ────
引き起こす 94
ひきずる 32
肥大 124
ぴったりとはめ込む 12
ひっぱる 32
ヒトゲノム 22
非薬物の 4
病気にかかった 32
標準誤差 80
病巣 126
病態生理学 55
病変 126
病歴 132
ピルビン酸塩 80

──── ふ ────
ファモチジン 113
フィトヘムアグルチニン ... 110
負荷 96
ふくらむ 12
付随する 127

147

負担 ……………… 96	〔精神的に〕麻痺させる …… 3	誘発する ………… 3, 95, 96
付着する ……………… 20	回す ……………… 80	有病率 ……………… 68
ブドウ糖 ……………… 69	慢性の ……………… 23	

─ よ ─

プラーク …………… 22, 32	─ み ─	用量依存性 …………… 79
プラセボ対照 ………… 81	ミオグロビン尿症 ……… 68	用量−作用効果 ………… 79
プロトコール ………… 79		溶血性貧血 …………… 119

─ へ ─

─ む ─

併発症状 …………… 131	無傷の ……………… 95	ヨガ ………………… 4
片頭痛 ……………… 3	無作為化 …………… 81	抑制する …………… 23
		予防 ………………… 55
		読み慣れた人 ………… 58
	─ め ─	弱められた ………… 87

─ ほ ─

傍正中の …………… 125	瞑想 ………………… 4	─ り ─
飽和脂肪 ………… 24, 25	眼の ……………… 125	
補助療法 …………… 20	免疫異常 …………… 119	罹患しやすくする …… 112
補体 ……………… 110	免疫蛍光法 ………… 119	離心性の …………… 125
発作 ………………… 2		両側性の …………… 109
ほとんど ………… 132	─ や ─	リン脂質 …………… 25
ホルモン …………… 14	薬物〔治療〕 …… 3, 4, 22	臨床医 …………… 131
翻訳された ………… 94		リンパ球減少 ……… 119
	─ ゆ ─	リンパ節炎 ………… 111

─ ま ─

毎日 ………………… 3	誘因 ……………… 3, 95, 96	─ れ ─
麻痺 ……………… 124	有害な ……………… 23	レーノー現象 ……… 109
	有機堆積物 ………… 23	

本書 Chapters 4〜6 で使用する音声教材，ならびに各 Chapter の Exercise の解答等をまとめた「教授用資料」を，ご希望の方にお分けします（ただし学校で授業の教材として利用されている学生の方は除きます）。ご希望の方は必ず<u>書面（FAX，E-mail も可）</u>にて，<u>書籍名・氏名・勤務先・送付先住所</u>を明記の上，下記へお申し込みください。

申込先：メジカルビュー社編集部　医学英語書籍担当者
〒162-0845 東京都新宿区市谷本村町 2-30
FAX　03-5228-2062
E-MAIL　ed@medicalview.co.jp

講義録　医学英語 I

（担当編集委員：清水雅子）

目次

Chapter 1	Characteristics of the Medical System in Japan
Chapter 2	Medical Terminology (1)
Chapter 3	Medical Terminology (2)
Chapter 4	Medical Terminology (3)
Chapter 5	Body Parts
Chapter 6	Listening to Medical News (1)
Chapter 7	Listening to Medical News (2)
Chapter 8	Listening to Medical News (3)
Chapter 9	Expressions to Describe Signs and Symptoms
Chapter 10	Expressions to Describe Vital Signs
Chapter 11	Expressions to Describe Pains
Chapter 12	Expressions to Use in the Examination

講義録　医学英語 III

（担当編集委員：J. Patrick Barron）

目次

Chapter 1	Learning Physical Examination (1)
Chapter 2	Learning Physical Examination (2)
Chapter 3	Learning Physical Examination (3)
Chapter 4	Learning Physical Examination (4)
Chapter 5	Giving an Oral Presentation (1)
Chapter 6	Giving an Oral Presentation (2)
Chapter 7	Giving an Oral Presentation (3)
Chapter 8	Writing the Medical Paper (1)
Chapter 9	Writing the Medical Paper (2)
Chapter 10	Writing the Medical Paper (3)

講義録

■体裁　B5 変型判，160 〜 850 頁程度，2 色刷り（一部カラー），定価 2,500 〜 9,000 円程度

呼吸器学
定価　5,775 円（5% 税込）　372 頁
- ◆編集　　杉山幸比古
- ◆編集協力　吉澤靖之，滝澤　始，吾妻安良太

循環器学
定価　6,300 円（5% 税込）　468 頁
- ◆編集　　小室一成
- ◆編集協力　川名正敏，萩原誠久，中村文隆，吉田勝哉

消化器学
定価　7,140 円（5% 税込）　700 頁
- ◆編集　上西紀夫，菅野健太郎，田中雅夫，滝川　一

内分泌・代謝学
定価　6,825 円（5% 税込）　548 頁
- ◆編集　寺本民生，片山茂裕

神経学
定価　7,140 円（5% 税込）　568 頁
- ◆編集　鈴木則宏，荒木信夫

腎臓学
定価　6,300 円（5% 税込）　400 頁
- ◆編集　木村健二郎，富野康日己

泌尿器学
定価　6,300 円（5% 税込）　352 頁
- ◆編集　荒井陽一，小川　修

眼・視覚学
定価　7,140 円（5% 税込）　384 頁（オールカラー）
- ◆編集　山本修一，大鹿哲郎

運動器学 第2版
定価 8,400円(5% 税込)　808頁
◆編集　三浪明男，戸山芳昭，越智光夫

小児科学
定価 8,925円(5% 税込)　808頁
◆編集　佐地　勉，有阪　治，大澤真木子，近藤直実，竹村　司

血液・造血器疾患学
定価 5,775円(5% 税込)　340頁
◆編集　小澤敬也，直江知樹，坂田洋一

腫瘍学
定価 5,250円(5% 税込)　240頁（オールカラー）
◆編集　高橋和久
◆編集協力　樋野興夫，齊藤光江，唐澤久美子

産科婦人科学
◆編集　石原　理，柴原浩章，三上幹男，板倉敦夫

医学英語Ⅰ　語彙の充実と読解力の向上　Building Vocabulary and Reading Comprehension
定価 2,625円(5% 税込)　168頁（教授用資料[12頁]，音声教材[CD 1枚]あり）
◆編集　日本医学英語教育学会 / 清水雅子

医学英語Ⅱ　科学英語への扉　Entering Scientific English in Context
定価 2,625円(5% 税込)　164頁（教授用資料[28頁]，音声教材[CD 1枚]あり）
◆編集　日本医学英語教育学会 / Nell L. Kennedy，蓑田治子

医学英語Ⅲ　専門英語の理解と実践　Principles and Practice of English for Medical Communications
定価 2,625円(5% 税込)　272頁（教授用資料[12頁]あり）
◆編集　日本医学英語教育学会 / J. Patrick Barron

メジカルビュー社

〒162-0845　東京都新宿区市谷本村町2番30号
TEL. 03-5228-2050　FAX. 03-5228-2059
URL http://www.medicalview.co.jp
E-mail（営業部）eigyo@medicalview.co.jp

講義録　医学英語Ⅱ　　科学英語への扉	
2005年12月20日　第1版第1刷発行	
2020年 2月10日　　　　　第8刷発行	

- ■編　集　日本医学英語教育学会
　　　　　　Nell L. Kennedy　　ネル・L・ケネディ
　　　　　　菱田治子　ひしだはるこ

- ■発行者　三澤　岳

- ■発行所　株式会社メジカルビュー社
　　　　　　〒162-0845 東京都新宿区市谷本村町2-30
　　　　　　電話　03(5228)2050(代表)
　　　　　　ホームページ http://www.medicalview.co.jp/

　　　　　　営業部　FAX 03(5228)2059
　　　　　　　　　　E-mail eigyo@medicalview.co.jp

　　　　　　編集部　FAX 03(5228)2062
　　　　　　　　　　E-mail ed@medicalview.co.jp

- ■印刷所　三美印刷株式会社

ISBN 978-4-7583-0408-5 C3347

© MEDICAL VIEW, 2005.　Printed in Japan

- ・本書に掲載された著作物の複写・複製・転載・翻訳・データベースへの取り込みおよび送信（送信可能化権を含む）・上映・譲渡に関する許諾権は，(株)メジカルビュー社が保有しています．

- ・JCOPY〈出版者著作権管理機構 委託出版物〉
本書の無断複製は著作権法上での例外を除き禁じられています．複製される場合は，そのつど事前に，出版者著作権管理機構（電話 03-5244-5088, FAX 03-5244-5089, e-mail：info@jcopy.or.jp）の許諾を得てください．

- ・本書をコピー，スキャン，デジタルデータ化するなどの複製を無許諾で行う行為は，著作権法上での限られた例外（「私的使用のための複製」など）を除き禁じられています．大学，病院，企業などにおいて，研究活動，診察を含み業務上使用する目的で上記の行為を行うことは私的使用には該当せず違法です．また私的使用のためであっても，代行業者等の第三者に依頼して上記の行為を行うことは違法となります．